Practical Guide to Gastroin
Function Testing

C000055073

Practical Guide to Gastrointestinal Function Testing

Charlotte Stendal MD

Medical Advisor
Medtronic GastroIntestinal
Synectics Medical AB
Renstiernas gata 12
S-11628 Stockholm
Sweden

Foreword by Dr Eamonn Quigley

**Blackwell
Science**

© Medtronic GastroIntestinal, 1997
All rights reserved

Published by
Blackwell Science Ltd
Editorial Offices:
Osney Mead, Oxford OX2 0EL
25 John Street, London WC1N 2BL
23 Ainslie Place, Edinburgh EH3 6AJ
350 Main Street, Malden
  MA 02148 5018, USA
54 University Street, Carlton
  Victoria 3053, Australia

Other Editorial Offices:
Blackwell Wissenschafts-Verlag GmbH
Kurfürstendamm 57
10707 Berlin, Germany

Blackwell Science KK
MG Kodenmacho Building
7–10 Kodenmacho Nihombashi
Chuo-ku, Tokyo 104, Japan

All rights reserved. No part of this
publication may be reproduced, stored in a
retrieval system, or transmitted, in any
form or by any means, electronic,
mechanical, photocopying, recording or
otherwise, except as permitted by the UK
Copyright, Designs and Patents Act 1988,
without the prior permission of the
copyright owner

First published 1997

Set by Alden Bookset Ltd
Printed and bound in the
United States of America by
Quebecor Printing, Tennessee

The Blackwell Science logo is a trade mark
of Blackwell Science Ltd, registered at the
United Kingdom Trade Marks Registry

DISTRIBUTORS

Marston Book Services Ltd
PO Box 269
Abingdon, Oxon OX14 4YN
(*Orders*: Tel: 01235 465500
          Fax: 01235 465555)

USA
  Blackwell Science, Inc.
  Commerce Place
  350 Main Street
  Malden, MA 02148 5018
  (*Orders*: Tel: 800 759 6102
                    617 388 8250
            Fax: 617 388 8255)

Canada
  Copp Clark Professional
  200 Adelaide St West, 3rd Floor
  Toronto, Ontario M5H 1W7
  (*Orders*: Tel: 416 597-1616
                    800 815-9417
            Fax: 416 597-1617)

Australia
  Blackwell Science Pty Ltd
  54 University Street
  Carlton, Victoria 3053
  (*Orders*: Tel: 3 9347 0300
            Fax: 3 9347 5001)

A catalogue record for this title
is available from the British Library

ISBN 0-632-04918-9

*The information in this guide is subject to
change without notice and should not be
construed as a commitment by Medtronic
GastroIntestinal. Medtronic
GastroIntestinal and the author assume no
responsibility for any error that may
appear in this book*

Contents

CONTENTS

Co-editors

Josephine D. Barlow BSc (HONS) FETC
Chief Clinical Gastrointestinal Physiologist, Hope Hospital, Salford, Manchester, UK

Guy E. Boeckxstaens MD PhD
*Division of Gastroenterology and Hepatology, Academic Medical Center,
Meibergdrief 9, 1105 AZ Amsterdam, Netherlands*

Cedric G. Bremner MB ChM FRCS(EDINBURGH) FACS
*University of Southern California School of Medicine, Department of Surgery,
Los Angeles, USA*

Tom R. DeMeester MD
*Professor and Chairman, Department of Surgery, University of Southern California,
Los Angeles, USA*

Ghislain Devroede
*Professor of Surgery and Communication, Faculty of Medicine, University of
Sherboorke, Quebec, Canada*

David Evans PhD
*Senior Lecturer and Research Coordinator, Gastrointestinal Science Research Unit,
St Bartholomew's and the Royal London School of Medicine and Dentistry,
University of London, UK*

Henrik Forsell MD PhD
Associate Professor, Department of Surgery, Blekinge Hospital, Karlskrona, Sweden

Karl H. Fuchs MD
Professor Dr, Department of Surgery, University of Wurzburg, Wurzburg, Germany

Peter Funch-Jensen MD DMSc
*Department of Surgical Gastroenterology, Hvidovre Hospital, University Hospital,
Hvidovre, Denmark*

Einar Husebye MD PhD
*Consultant in Gastroenterology, Clinic of Medicine, Ullevaal University Hospital of
Oslo, Norway*

CO-EDITORS

Peter Milla MSc MRCP
Reader in Paediatric Gastroenterology and Nutrition, Institute of Child Health,
University College London, UK

William C. Orr PhD
President and Chief Operating Officer, Institute for Healthcare Research,
Baptist Medical Center of Oklahoma, USA

Sandro Passaretti MD
Senior Registrar, Gastroenterology and Gastrointestinal Endoscopy Unit,
San Raffaele Hospital, 20132 Milano, Italy

Eamonn M. M. Quigley MD FRCP
Associate Professor of Medicine, Chief, Section of Gastroenterology and Hepatology,
University of Nebraska Medical Center, Omaha, USA

Joel Richter MD
Chairman, The Cleveland Clinic Foundation, Department of Gastroenterology,
Cleveland, Ohio, USA

Manfred Ritter MD
Dr, Department of Surgery, University of Wurzburg, Wurzburg, Germany

Yvan Vandenplas MD PhD
Head of Paediatrics, Academic Childrens Hospital, Brussels, Belgium

Foreword

Recent years have witnessed tremendous progress in the field of gastro-intestinal (GI) motility. Advances in our understanding of the generation and modulation of motor events throughout the GI tract has been greatly increased by progress in basic and applied science. We have come to appreciate the complex interactions between GI smooth muscle, the enteric nervous system, autonomic nerves and the central nervous system. The role of gut sensation is now appreciated, and the importance of interactions between the gut and the brain, as well as between various parts of the GI tract, increasingly emphasized. As the science of motility has flourished, our appreciation of the clinical importance of this field has grown apace. Disorders based on motor dysfunction or where dysmotility is, at the very least, a contributing factor, are recognized as commonplace and responsible for considerable morbidity. Such disorders have also, traditionally, pre-sented formidable diagnostic and therapeutic challenges.

For years, the practising clinician had a relatively restricted armamen-tarium available for the assessment of these putative motility disorders. Diagnostic efforts were often confined to relatively subjective, qualitative descriptions of motor patterns. The past several years have witnessed a veritable revolution in the field of motility diagnostics. Taking advantage of tremendous advances in the miniaturization of sensors, computer soft-ware and display systems, a wide variety of highly sophisticated diagnostic methodologies are at our disposal. The clinician can now record intra-luminal pressure activity from virtually any part of the GI tract, and often from multiple sites over prolonged periods of time, if this is desired. The resultant signals are digitized, analyzed and displayed in a readily interpre-table manner, and can be easily subjected to a variety of statistical manipu-lations. Luminal phenomena, such as pH and bilirubin concentration, can be monitored over time and correlated with symptomatology. Most recently, techniques for the objective assessment of tone, compliance and sensation in various parts of the GI tract have been introduced and have already exerted a significant impact on clinical research. In some areas, manometric and fluoroscopic images can now be displayed simultaneously and correlated directly. These new technologies have also been used in the area of therapeutics—for example, manometric and electromyographic signals are already used to guide biofeedback therapy.

Engineers and computer scientists have opened the Pandora's Box—it is our task as clinicians and investigators to employ these tools for the optimum benefit of our patients. This must involve the appropriate and judicious use of available technology to truly advance diagnosis and guide therapy. Technology must not be employed for its own sake, but rather, for that of our patients' well being.

This book serves to introduce a range of technologies which may be used in the assessment of GI motor disorders. While a critical evaluation of the indications and interpretation of each of these modalities, in all situations where they may be utilized, is beyond the scope of this volume, each will be discussed in an appropriate clinical context, and some general guides for their use outlined. The emphasis, however, will be on helping the neophyte as well as the experienced investigator to establish the technique in their laboratory, to optimize its use and troubleshoot problems.

We hope that you will find this book a useful introduction to the clinical study of GI motility and its disorders, and that it will help promote the evaluation, and further the management of these challenging disorders.

Eamonn Quigley

Preface

The investigation of gastrointestinal (GI) diseases has changed enormously over recent decades. The alimentary tract used to be a dark and impenetrable region beyond the reach of physicians. Then fibreoptic endoscopy shed light on the gut and gastroenterologists had the luxury of being able to see what the problem was. Or did they? Some disorders of the GI system cannot be diagnosed visually, most notably disorders of motility.

In recent years an enormous amount of research into GI physiology has yielded a plethora of new techniques, such as pH monitoring, manometry and more recently electrogastrography. These have now become common methods for investigating GI diseases around the world.

The techniques are, however, only as good as the clinicians and clinical scientists that use them. This book is intended as a practical guide that will enable any GI centre to select the most appropriate tests for any suspected disorder, and then gives step-by-step descriptions of how to perform the procedure.

Many of the tests described require a basic knowledge of the anatomy of the GI tract. An introductory chapter is intended to refresh the dim and distant recollections of anatomy, and places this within a clinical context. The next four chapters adopt a problem-solving approach to disorders in each major region of the digestive system. Each disease is described under consistently applied headings, for ease of reference, and the most appropriate diagnostic procedures are highlighted.

The procedures themselves are described in Chapter 8. Again I have used consistent headings (indications; contraindications; equipment; before the study; during the study; procedure; after the study; interpretation; pitfalls) so that the reader can find information quickly and use this section as a bench manual.

There are also two chapters that the reader might be surprised to find in a book of this type. These focus on pediatric GI disease. Children present special problems for diagnosis and the techniques described in this book are a useful way of "quantifying" a disorder that a child might have difficulty describing. In some cases the techniques need significant modification, while in others they are pretty much the same as those used in adults.

PREFACE

This book has been the product of many years' work. It would have been impossible without the help of a number of highly motivated, and extremely busy clinical investigators who have critically read all that I have included in this book. I am tremendously grateful to these contributing co-editors, who have been listed on p. vii. I would especially like to thank Dr Eamonn Quigley who, as well as taking time to carefully review the manuscript, also wrote the Foreword to this text. Thank you also to Dr Manfred Ritter for writing the section on the Ambulatory Counter, and Mr Jonas Zaar for supplying the original illustrations.

Charlotte Stendal

Abbreviations

CIIP	Chronic idiopathic intestinal pseudoobstruction
CIP	Chronic intestinal pseudoobstruction
CPM	Cycles per minute
DES	Diffuse esophageal spasm
DGER	Duodeno-gastro-esophageal reflux
EAS	External anal sphincter
EGG	Electrogastrography
EMG	Electromyography
ENS	Enteric nervous system
ERCP	Endoscopic retrograde cholangiopancreatography
GER	Gastroesophageal reflux
GERD	Gastroesophageal reflux disease
GI	Gastrointestinal
HAPC	High amplitude propagated contractions
HPZ	High pressure zone
IAS	Internal anal sphincter
IBS	Irritable bowel syndrome
IHD	Ischemic heart disease
LES	Lower esophageal sphincter
NCCP	Noncardiac chest pain
NEMD	Nonspecific esophageal motility disorders
MMC	Migrating motor complex
PIP	Pressure inversion point
RAIR	Rectoanal inhibitory reflex
RMC	Rectal motor complex
RIP	Respiratory inversion point
SO	Sphincter of Oddi
SPT	Station pull through
SLE	Systemic lupus erythematosus
TLESR	Transient lower esophageal sphincter relaxation
UES	Upper esophageal sphincter

1 Anatomy of the Digestive System

Simplistically, the gastrointestinal (GI) tract is a series of hollow organs joined in a muscled tube from the mouth to the anus. Depending on the different diameters of the tube and the different characteristic functions, it can be divided into the following sections:

- esophagus
- stomach
- small bowel
- colon
- rectum
- anus.

There are also two solid digestive organs, the liver and the pancreas, which produce juices that reach the intestines through small tubes (Fig. 1.1).

The purpose of the digestive system is to digest food—the process of breaking down food and fluids into their smallest components, so that the body can use them for building and nourishing cells and providing energy.

1.1 Basic wall structure of the gastrointestinal tract

The walls of the entire digestive tract are organized into a number of distinct layers. They consist of the following (Fig. 1.2).

Mucosa

The mucosa is the inner coating of the hollow organs. It separates the luminal contents of the gut from the internal compartments of the bowel wall. It is composed of an epithelial lining, a lamina propria and a muscularis mucosa.

In the esophagus and the distal portion of the anal canal the epithelial lining consists of squamous epithelium. In the rest of the digestive tract it is made up of columnar epithelial cells. The organization of these cells, however, is different in each organ.

Below the epithelial lining, within the lamina propria there is a network of blood, lymph vessels, and the immunocytes of the gut-associated lymphoid tissue, which is an important first line of defense against pathogens.

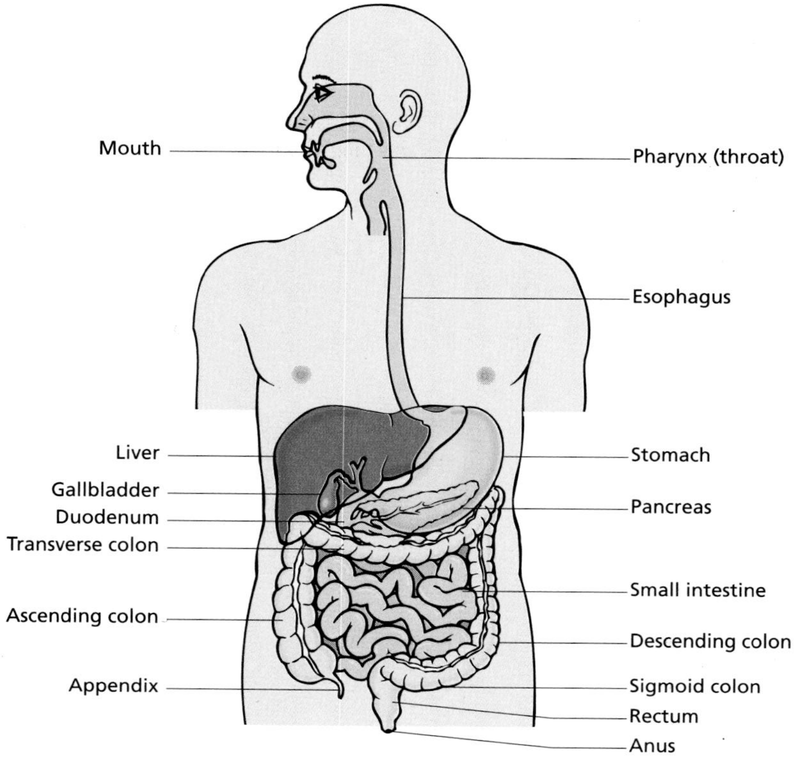

Mouth

Pharynx (throat)

Esophagus

Liver

Stomach

Gallbladder

Duodenum

Pancreas

Transverse colon

Ascending colon

Small intestine

Descending colon

Appendix

Sigmoid colon

Rectum

Anus

Figure 1.1 The digestive system.

Submucosa

The submucosa is the layer below the mucosa. A thin sheet of muscle, the muscularis mucosae, separates the mucosa and submucosa. The submucosa contains blood and lymph vessels, and a nerve network called the submucosal plexus (Meissner's plexus). In the esophagus it also contains glands that produce mucus.

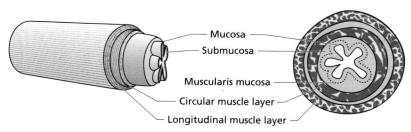

Mucosa

Submucosa

Muscularis mucosa

Circular muscle layer

Longitudinal muscle layer

Figure 1.2 Drawing of the esophagus showing the basic wall structure of the GI tract.

Muscle layer

The muscle of the gut wall consists of muscle fibers which are organized into a number of layers. The muscle fibers in each layer are arranged in a different direction. Most digestive organs have two muscle layers, an inner circular and an outer longitudinal. The stomach is one exception, having an additional oblique layer, and the colon is another since the outer longitudinal layer is organized into three discrete bands of muscles which run along the length of the colon (the taenia coli).

A nerve network called the myenteric plexus (Auerbach's plexus) is located between the circular and longitudinal muscle layers.

With only two exceptions, the muscle fibers which make up the muscle layer of the GI tract consist of smooth muscle fibers. The muscle layer of the proximal part of the esophagus including the upper esophageal sphincter (UES) and the distal anal canal with its external anal sphincter are made up of striated muscle fibers.

Outer cover/serosa

The serosa, a layer of connective tissue, forms the external lining of the digestive organs. For the stomach and the intestines the serosa is continuous with the peritoneum (a serous membranous covering).

1.2 Neural regulation of gastrointestinal motility

The neural regulation of the digestive system is very complex and largely beyond our conscious control. However, the proximal end of the esophagus and the anus are exceptions. The muscle layers here consist of striated muscle fibers which are to some extent under voluntary control. The neural regulation of the rest of the digestive tract is provided by the autonomic nervous system (sympathetic and parasympathetic nerves) and the enteric nervous system (ENS) (a network of nerve cells and their connections in the gut wall).

The neural innervation of the GI tract can be divided into extrinsic and intrinsic components (Fig. 1.3).

Extrinsic innervation

Extrinsic innervation is provided either by somatic motor nerves or by the autonomic nervous system (Fig. 1.4).

SOMATIC MOTOR INNERVATION

The motor innervation of the striated muscles in the pharynx and proximal esophagus is provided mainly via the motor components of the lower cranial nerves.

Motor innervation of the striated muscles in the anal canal is mainly provided by the pudendal nerve.

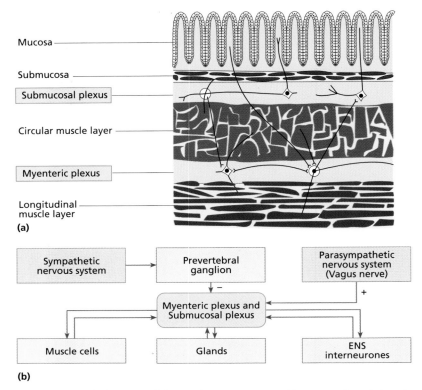

Mucosa

Submucosa

Submucosal plexus

Circular muscle layer

Myenteric plexus

Longitudinal muscle layer

(a)

| Sympathetic nervous system | → | Prevertebral ganglion | | Parasympathetic nervous system (Vagus nerve) |

Myenteric plexus and Submucosal plexus

| Muscle cells | | Glands | | ENS interneurones |

(b)

Figure 1.3 (a) The location of the enteric nervous system (the myenteric and the submucosal plexus). (b) Shows the myenteric and submucosal plexus working as relay neurons for the sympathetic and parasympathetic system.

AUTONOMIC INNERVATION

The majority of the GI tract is under autonomic control (controlled without our conscious control). The autonomic nervous system is divided into two parts:

- The *parasympathetic* nervous system, which includes the vagus nerve, acts primarily to stimulate GI motility. Even though many different neurotransmitters are involved, acetylcholine is considered the most important neurotransmitter to stimulate smooth muscle activity and hormonal systems. The parasympathetic nervous system uses the myenteric plexus (see below) as relay neurons
- The *sympathetic* nervous system acts mainly to decrease GI activity. Its nerves reach the myenteric plexus (see below) via a series of ganglia. Norepinephrine is the most important neurotransmitter in the sympathetic system.

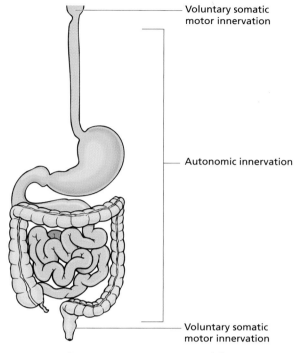

Figure 1.4 Autonomic and somatic motor innervation of the GI tract.

Intrinsic innervation

Intrinsic innervation of the GI tract is provided by the ENS, a complex and highly sophisticated internal regulator for the modification of GI motility.

The motor activity of the GI tract is mainly generated by the activity of the ENS. It receives afferent messages directly from the gut and can rapidly generate appropriate response with or without involving the autonomic nervous system. The ENS is therefore often referred to as "the little brain of the gut."

The nerves of the ENS are also considered as the relay neurons between parasympathetic and sympathetic nerves, and smooth muscle cells, the glands of the gut mucosa, and other intramural nerve cells. In this way the autonomic nervous system, or indeed the central nervous system can modulate the activity of the ENS.

The ENS consists of two different nerve networks:
- the myenteric plexus (Auerbach's plexus) which is the nerve network located between the circular and longitudinal muscular layers
- the submucosal plexus (Meissner's plexus) which is a nerve network located in the submucosa, between the mucosa and the circular muscle layer.

1.3 Hormonal regulation of gastrointestinal motility

Motility and sphincter pressures in the GI tract are also regulated by many of the hormones secreted by the digestive tract (Table 1.1).

Table 1.1 Hormones of the digestive tract.

Hormone	Origin	Action
Gastrin	Antrum	Increases LES pressure, stimulates motility in the small bowel and gallbladder
CCK	Duodenum and jejunum	Stimulates contraction of the gallbladder. Slows emptying of the stomach and reduces small bowel motility
Secretin	Duodenal and jejunal mucosa	Inhibits emptying of the stomach by increasing pressure in the pylorus. Inhibitory effect on the small bowel and large intestine
Motilin	Duodenum	Accelerates gastric emptying. Modulates the migrating motor complexes
Somatostatin	Pancreas (islets of Langerhans) and hypothalamus	Inhibits many GI secretions. Role in motility unclear. Increases gastric emptying after liquid meals
GIP	Mucosa in the upper small intestine	Slows gastric emptying when bowel is full

CCK, cholecystokinin; GIP, gastric inhibitory peptide; LES, lower esophageal sphincter.

1.4 Esophagus

The main purpose of the esophagus is to transport food to the stomach. It consists of a muscular tube, approximately 25 cm long, with sphincters, the upper esophageal sphincter (UES) and the lower esophageal sphincter (LES) at either end. The sphincters help to keep the esophagus empty between swallows while also preventing regurgitation of stomach contents to the esophagus, larynx, and the oral cavity.

The esophagus narrows somewhat at three levels (Fig. 1.5):
- the UES
- the middle section where the aorta and left bronchi press against the esophagus
- the point at which the esophagus passes through the diaphragm.

Foreign bodies such as food, etc., are more likely to get stuck at each of these points.

The upper esophageal sphincter

The UES is formed by the cricopharyngeus muscle. It forms a loop around the upper end of the esophagus and attaches to the cricoid cartilage. The circular muscle sublayer of the esophagus is also continuous with the UES.

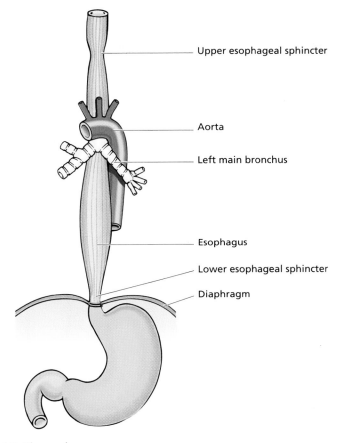

Figure 1.5 The esophagus.

The upper sphincter is of great importance in preventing regurgitation of esophageal contents to the oral cavity and the larynx, and thereby protecting against choking and aspiration.

The lower esophageal sphincter

The LES is composed of smooth muscle. It is usually located at the level of the diaphragm where the esophagus passes from the thoracic into the abdominal cavity. By maintaining a high pressure zone between the stomach and the esophagus, the LES is of primary importance in preventing the reflux of gastric contents from the stomach.

The esophageal wall

The esophageal wall is 3–4 mm thick. Similar to the walls in the entire digestive tract, it consists of four main layers (Fig. 1.6).

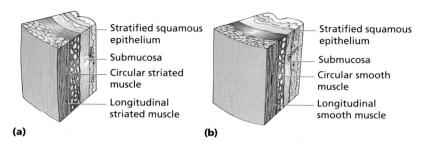

(a)
- Stratified squamous epithelium
- Submucosa
- Circular striated muscle
- Longitudinal striated muscle

(b)
- Stratified squamous epithelium
- Submucosa
- Circular smooth muscle
- Longitudinal smooth muscle

Figure 1.6 Section of the esophageal wall. (a) Proximal part with striated muscle layers and (b) distal part with smooth muscle layers.

MUCOSA

The mucosa, which is the inner coating of the esophagus, consists of squamous epithelial cells which extends to the Z-line where it abruptly converts to the columnar epithelium of the stomach. The Z-line which runs circumferentially in a somewhat zig-zag fashion represents the demarcation between the gastric and the esophageal mucosa. In normal individuals the Z-line or squamous–columnar junction occurs at the level of the LES (approximately 2 cm proximal to the anatomical borderline between the esophagus and the cardia of the stomach).

SUBMUCOSA

The submucosa consists of collagen and elastic fibers. It contains glands that produce mucus, which functions as a protective film and lubricant in the esophagus.

MUSCLE LAYER

The muscles of the esophageal wall are organized into two layers: an inner circular and an outer longitudinal layer. This arrangement of muscle fibers facilitates peristaltic contractions and the transit of luminal contents into the stomach.

The muscle fibers that make up the muscular layers in the esophagus are of two types (Fig. 1.7):
- Striated muscle fibers make up the proximal third of the esophagus and the UES. Although this part of the esophagus consists of striated muscle fibers, its voluntary control is limited (e.g. the initiation of a swallow). For the most part, it is under autonomic control
- Smooth muscle fibers. As one moves toward the distal esophagus the wall consists of an increasing number of smooth muscle fibers. The distal third of the esophagus consists of smooth muscle fibers alone. These fibers are completely controlled by the enteric and autonomic nervous systems.

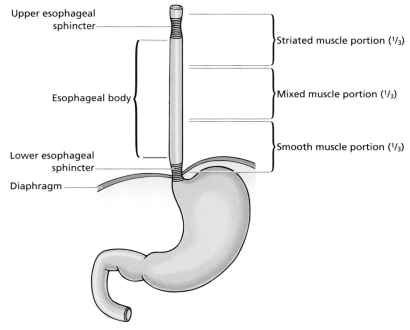

Figure 1.7 The esophageal body illustrating striated and smooth muscle portions.

OUTER COVERING

In the thoracic part of the esophagus the outer cover consists of connective tissue which is elastic and can stretch as the esophagus distends during the passage of food. In the abdominal part, after passing through the diaphragm, the esophagus is surrounded by the peritoneum.

Innervation

- The motor innervation of the striated muscles in the proximal esophagus is provided via motor nerves in the vagus nerve which originates in the brainstem. Each motor nerve fiber ends directly on several striated muscle fibers which it directly activates (Fig. 1.8)
- The autonomic innervation of the smooth muscle in the distal esophagus occurs via the parasympathetic and sympathetic nervous systems. All parasympathetic input to the esophagus is provided via the vagus nerve.

ENTERIC INNERVATION

The myenteric plexus (Auerbach's plexus) controls motor activities of the muscular layer. This nerve network is located between the circular and longitudinal muscular layers of the esophagus. The submucosal plexus is sparse in the esophagus (see Fig. 1.3).

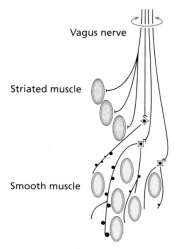

Figure 1.8 Motor nerves end directly on several striated muscle fibers.

1.5 Stomach

The capacity of the human stomach is variable. In basal conditions it contains 200–300 ml, but can increase its capacity to contain as much as 1–1.5 l. It has five main functions:

1 as a food reservoir
2 to mix and grind food
3 to chemically break down food
4 to kill ingested microbes
5 to control emptying of gastric contents into the duodenum.

The stomach is divided up into different sections (Fig. 1.9):

• The cardia joins the stomach and the esophagus

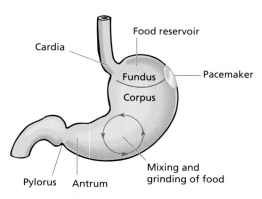

Figure 1.9 The stomach and its different parts.

- The fundus is the upper section under the left part of the diaphragm. This is where ingested food is received. It is also the main food reservoir
- The corpus is the largest section of the stomach. Hydrochloric acid (HCl) and the enzyme pepsin are produced here as well as in the fundus. The pacemaker area of the stomach is located on the greater curvature of the corpus. The electrical impulses which generate gastric peristalsis are initiated at this site
- The antrum is the section where the hormone gastrin is produced. There is no acid secretion (HCl) in this section but the hormone gastrin is secreted into the bloodstream and stimulates acid production by parietal cells in the corpus of the stomach. The antrum is also the pincipal site where the solid food particles are ground down before they are emptied into the duodenum
- The pylorus is the sphincter between the stomach and the duodenum. It controls the emptying of food into the duodenum, and also limits regurgitation of duodenal contents back into the stomach.

The gastric wall
This consists of the following.

MUCOSA
The mucosa, consisting of columnar epithelium, is organized into longitudinal folds called plicae (Fig. 1.10). This arrangement greatly increases the surface area of the gastric mucosa and thereby promotes the exposure of the contents of the stomach to the stomach wall.

Digestive juices are secreted by gastric glands (Fig. 1.11) covering nearly the entire surface of the stomach's corpus. The glands consist of:

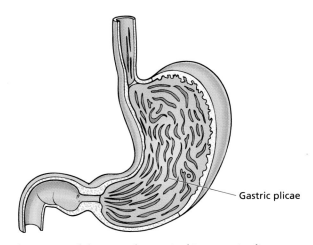

Gastric plicae

Figure 1.10 The mucosa of the stomach organized into gastric plicae.

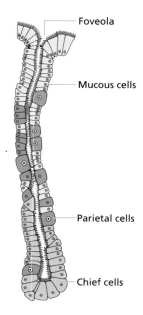

Figure 1.11 The gastric gland.

- mucous cells that produce a mucus layer which protects the stomach against digestion by gastric secretions
- parietal cells that produce HCl and intrinsic factor
- chief cells that produce pepsinogen.

The glandular tubules terminate in microscopic pits called foveolae.

MUSCLE LAYERS (Fig. 1.12)

The muscular layer of the stomach differs from that of the rest of the GI tract. It consists of smooth muscle fibers organized into three different

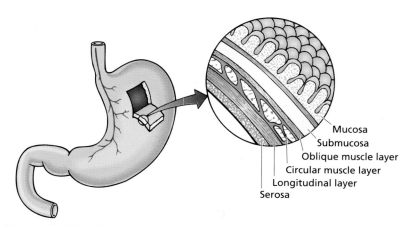

Figure 1.12 The wall of the stomach.

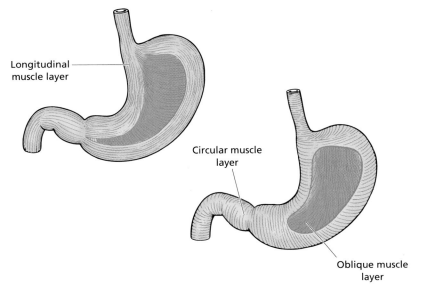

Longitudinal muscle layer

Circular muscle layer

Oblique muscle layer

Figure 1.13 There are three muscle layers of the stomach: longitudinal, circular, and oblique.

muscular layers. The fibers in each layer are arranged in different directions: longitudinal, circular, and an additional inner oblique layer (Fig. 1.13).

The muscles of the stomach are arranged to provide the most efficient grinding and mixing of food. The oblique layer facilitates receptive relaxation on meal ingestion; a phenomenon necessary for the reservoir function of the stomach. However, at the cardia and pyloric sphincter, a circular orientation of smooth muscle fibers predominates to facilitate sphincteric action.

OUTER COVERING

The serosa which forms the outer lining of the stomach is continuous with the peritoneum except along the greater and lesser curvatures where it connects with the omentum.

INNERVATION

The extrinsic innervation of the stomach is autonomic.

- The parasympathetic nervous system via the vagus nerve (Fig. 1.14) mainly stimulates smooth muscle activity and increases the motility and secretion of the gut. However, in the fundus of the stomach the vagal activity causes receptive relaxation on food intake
- The sympathetic nervous system has the opposite function and mainly decreases the activity of the smooth muscles by either reducing neurotransmitter release from cholinergic neurons or by acting directly on smooth muscle cells.

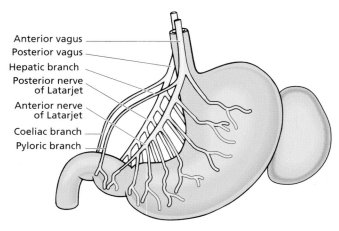

Figure 1.14 The vagus nerve.

The intrinsic innervation of the stomach is provided by the ENS including the myenteric and submucosal plexus.

There are also many different hormones from the digestive tract that regulate stomach activity (see Table 1.1).

1.6 Small bowel

The role of the small bowel is to digest and absorb nutrients. Digestion is the breakdown of the three major macronutrients (carbohydrates, proteins, and fat) into absorbable components.

The movements of the small bowel serve to:
1 mix the food with the digestive juices
2 make digestive products come in contact with the digestive–absorptive surface of the small intestine
3 propel waste products to the colon.
The small bowel is approximately 3–5 m long. It is made up of three different sections: the duodenum, jejunum, and ileum.

Duodenum

The duodenum is the shortest part of the small bowel. It starts at the pylorus and forms a C-shape around the head of the pancreas down to the jejunum (Fig. 1.15). The ligament of Treitz, which anchors the distal part of the duodenum, is often used as an anatomic landmark when positioning antroduodenal probes.

The beginning of the duodenum, the duodenal bulb, is slightly wider than the rest, and is approximately 3–4 cm wide.

Bile and pancreatic juices empty into the duodenum via the common bile and pancreatic ducts. These ducts unite in the wall of the duodenum to form

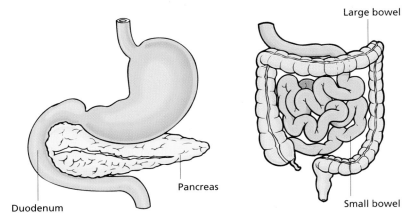

Figure 1.15 Position of the duodenum and the small bowel.

a common channel, the ampulla of Vater, which is surrounded by a ring of circular muscle—the sphincter of Oddi.

Jejunum and ileum

Beyond the duodenum the small bowel continues as the jejunum and the ileum. There is no strict border between the jejunum and the ileum. Approximately three-fifths of the small bowel is considered to be the ileum. The mucosa of the jejunum, however, is folded somewhat more than the mucosa of the ileum.

The wall of the small intestine

The wall of the small intestine is organized into layers identical to the rest of the digestive system (Fig. 1.16).

MUCOSA

The mucosa consists of columnar epithelial cells. The surface area of the mucosa is dramatically increased firstly by its arrangement into circular folds, plicae circulares; secondly, by the presence of projections, the intestinal villi; and finally, the presence of microvilli on the surface of each epithelial cell. This arrangement increases surface area more than 500-fold.

This provides a large enough surface for the absorption of digestive products. In between the villi are depressions, or crypts, which contain glands which secrete mucus and digestive juices. There are also specialized epithelial cells which secrete hormones (see Table 1.1).

Lymphoid tissue is plentiful in the small intestine and in some areas is organized into discrete aggregations referred to as Peyer's patches.

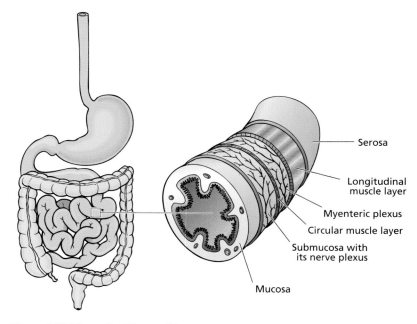

Figure 1.16 The wall of the small bowel.

SUBMUCOSA

The submucosa is a mobile layer of connective tissue that includes the submucosal nerve plexus and the major networks of blood and lymph vessels.

MUSCLE LAYER

The muscle layer consists of an inner circular and an outer longitudinal layer. The longitudinal muscle shortens and dilates the relevant portion of the intestine, whereas the circular muscle layer narrows and elongates the intestine.

The myenteric plexus is located between the muscle layers and coordinates motor activity of the small bowel in order to propel contents distally (Fig. 1.17).

OUTER COVERING

The serosa which forms the outer cover of the jejunum and the ileum is entirely continuous with the peritoneum. The duodenum, however, lies behind the peritoneum.

MOTILITY

Motility in the small bowel is controlled by:
- the autonomic nervous system including the sympathetic and parasympathetic systems

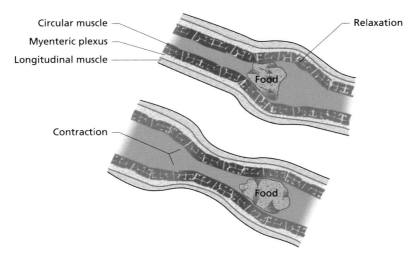

Circular muscle
Myenteric plexus
Longitudinal muscle
Relaxation
Food

Contraction
Food

Figure 1.17 A peristaltic contraction of the small bowel which propels contents distally. Longitudinal muscle shortens and dilates and circular muscle narrows and elongates the segment of the intestine.

- the ENS including the myenteric and submucosal plexus
- hormones (see Table 1.1).

1.7 Colon—the large bowel (Fig. 1.18)

The main purpose of the colon is to:
1 absorb water and electrolytes which have entered the intestine with the digestive juices
2 transport waste products
3 temporarily store waste products.

The colon is approximately 1.3 m long and consists of:
- cecum with its appendix. The distal part of the ileum protrudes into the cecum as a round or oval papilliform projection. This is called the ileocecal valve
- ascending colon
- transverse colon
- descending colon
- sigmoid colon.

The wall of the large bowel

MUCOSA

The mucosa, which has a fairly smooth surface, is organized into semicircular folds, the plica semilunares. The mucosa consists of a single layer of tall columnar epithelial cells. There are no villi in the colon, but there are crypts

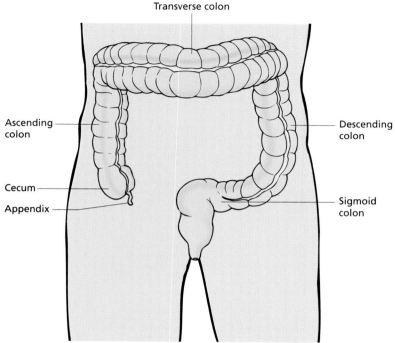

Figure 1.18 The large bowel—colon.

where the epithelium consists almost entirely of goblet cells which produce lubricating mucus. As in the small intestine, there are lymphatic glands.

MUSCLE LAYER

The muscle layer is organized into an inner circular and an outer longitudinal layer (Fig. 1.19). The outer, longitudinal, layer is not circumferential in the colon but is instead organized into three bands of muscle groups, called the taenia coli.

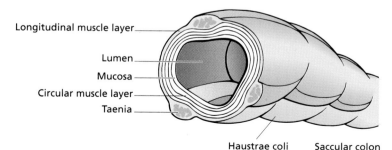

Figure 1.19 Muscular arrangement in the colon. Contractions of the smooth circular muscle creates the form of haustra.

OUTER COVERING

The serosa of the ascending and descending colon lie partly behind the peritoneum, i.e. continuous with the peritoneum on the front only. The transverse and the sigmoid colon lie within the peritoneum. The cecum is sometimes covered with the peritoneum but can also be fixed to the posterior wall of the trunk behind the peritoneum.

INNERVATION

- Autonomic nervous system
- Enteric nervous system. Intrinsic innervation via the myenteric and submucosal plexus.

1.8 Rectum

The rectum is continuous with the sigmoid colon and begins at the level of the third sacral vertebra. It is S-shaped and follows the curvature of the sacrum and coccyx for its entire length of approximately 15 cm. It has three lateral curves and the inner aspects of these transverse folds are called the rectal valves of Houston (Fig. 1.20).

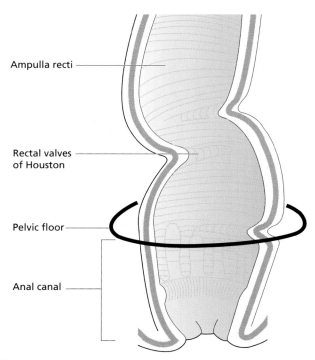

Ampulla recti

Rectal valves of Houston

Pelvic floor

Anal canal

Figure 1.20 Section through the rectum and the anal canal.

Ampulla recti

The ampulla recti refers to the upper part of the rectum. Normally, this part is completely empty of fecal material. The fecal material is stored in the sigmoid colon, but when fecal material reaches the ampulla recti, the sensation of the urge to defecate is initiated.

Pelvic floor

The rectum passes down through the pelvic floor which consists of musculotendinous sheets composed predominantly of striated fibers known as the levator ani muscles.

As the rectum passes through the pelvis to join the anal canal, its course is not straight as its name suggests, but forms an angle of approximately 90° (Fig. 1.21). This angle is of great importance in the maintenance of fecal continence.

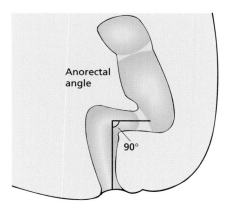

Anorectal angle

90°

Figure 1.21 The anorectal angle.

1.9 Anal canal

The pelvic floor forms the border between the rectum and the anal canal. The anal canal is approximateyly 3–4 cm long and is surrounded by sphincter muscles (Fig. 1.22).

The anal canal wall

This is organized into the following layers.

MUCOSA

The upper part of the canal is lined by columnar epithelium.

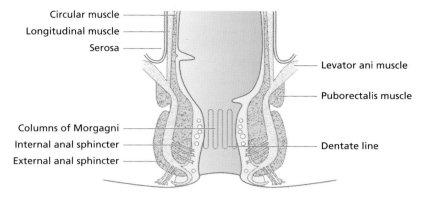

Circular muscle
Longitudinal muscle
Serosa
Levator ani muscle
Puborectalis muscle
Columns of Morgagni
Internal anal sphincter
External anal sphincter
Dentate line

Figure 1.22 Longitudinal section of the anal canal.

The distal portion of the anal canal is lined by anoderm, a thin layer of stratified squamous epithelium that lacks sweat glands and hair follicles. The border between these epithelia is called the linea mucocutanea or dentate line.

Several longitudinal mucosal folds (the columnae anales or the columns of Morgagni) arise in the proximal anal canal and terminate at the dentate line, where they surround the anal crypts with tubular anal glands. The mucosa here has a purple appearance compared to the pink color of the rest of the mucosa in the anal canal. The reason for this is that the mucosa overlies three vascular anal cushions often referred to as internal hemorrhoids.

Outer hemorrhoids are located in the venous plexa in the mucocutaneous border in the anus.

MUSCULAR LAYER

There are two sphincters, the internal anal sphincter and the external anal sphincter, which together with the pelvic floor work as holding forces to maintain fecal continence.

Internal sphincter

The internal sphincter is a continuation of the inner circular smooth muscle layer of the rectum and maintains a continuous muscle tone which demonstrates cyclic fluctuations. It is totally under autonomic control and is mainly responsible for the resting pressure of the anal canal.

External sphincter

The external sphincter is usually divided into three parts: the subcutaneous, superficial, and deep parts.

The external sphincter is responsible for the pressure on voluntary squeeze but also contributes to the resting pressure. The external sphincter consists of two different types of striated muscle fibers, red and white. Even though the red muscle fibers appear to be voluntary, they can maintain a state of tonic contraction in much the same manner as the internal sphincter. The white fibers are capable of powerful contractions but can only maintain this maximal contraction level for a short time.

Levator ani muscle

The levator ani muscle in the pelvic floor consists of the pubococcygeus (with the puborectalis muscle forming the puborectal sling (Fig. 1.23)), ileococcygeus, and ischiococcygeus; however, variations exist. The puborectalis muscle is especially important since the contraction of this muscle maintains the anorectal angle at approximately 90°. This angle is of great functional importance in the maintenance of continence (see Fig. 1.21).

INNERVATION

The rectum and the upper part of the anal canal are innervated by fibers from the autonomic and the enteric nervous systems (Fig. 1.24).

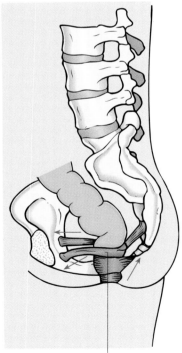

Puborectal sling

Figure 1.23 Puborectal sling.

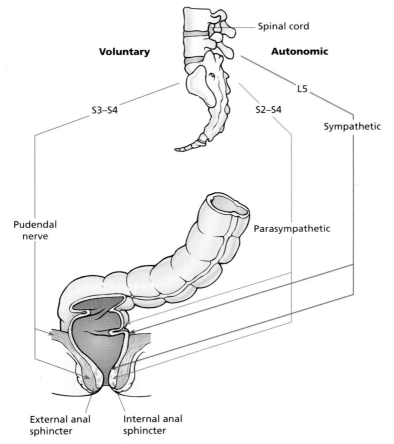

Figure 1.24 Innervation of the anorectal region.

The external sphincter and the levator ani muscles are innervated by somatic nerves. Branches arise from the 2nd, 3rd, and 4th sacral nerves and join the pudendal nerve. The puborectalis muscle also receives a direct branch from S3–S4.

The sensation to the perianal region and anal canal, distal to the dentate line, is conveyed by afferent fibers of the inferior rectal nerves. The mucosa of the rectum and proximal anal canal lack somatic sensory innervation.

1.10 Gallbladder (Fig. 1.25)

The functions of the gallbladder are to:
1 work as a bile reservoir
2 concentrate the bile by absorbing water.
The oval-shaped gallbladder has an average volume of approximately 20 ml of bile juice.

23

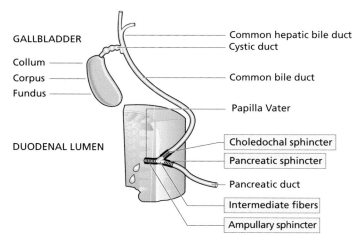

Figure 1.25 Macroscopic structure of the gallbladder, major bile ducts, and the sphincter of Oddi with its different parts.

Bile reaches the gallbladder via the cystic duct from the common hepatic bile duct originating in the liver.

Bile empties mainly in relation to meals, in response to hormones released by the duodenum, and is then transported to the duodenum via the cystic duct and the common bile duct.

The main purpose of bile is to emulsify fats in the lumen so they can be absorbed.

The pancreatic duct is usually united with the common bile duct to form the ampulla of Vater that empties into the duodenum.

There are, however, considerable anatomical variations in this area. Either the pancreatic and common bile duct merge together to a common channel or join without a common duct at the orifice of the ampulla of Vater. The ducts may also have entirely separate openings into the duodenum.

As the ducts pass through the wall of the duodenum they are surrounded by a distinct ring of circular muscle (a thickening of the smooth muscle layer), the sphincter of Oddi.

Sphincter of Oddi

The sphincter of Oddi can be subdivided into different parts (see Fig. 1.25):
- choledochal sphincter
- pancreatic sphincter
- ampullary sphincter
- intermediate fibers (between the sphincter segments listed above).

The sphincter of Oddi is a unique high pressure zone with superimposed phasic activity to regulate the flow of pancreatic juice and bile into the duodenum.

1.11 Pancreas (Fig. 1.26)

The pancreas is composed of several different types of cells with two main functions:

1 exocrine function: the secretion of digestive juices (pancreatic juice) from the acini
2 endocrine function: the production of insulin, glucagon, and somatostatin from the islets of Langerhans.

Pancreatic juice contains:
- enzymes for digesting protein, carbohydrate, and fat
- bicarbonate ions and water to neutralize acid emptied into the duodenum from the stomach.

The pancreas is made up of three parts:
- caput (head of the pancreas)
- corpus (body)
- cauda (tail).

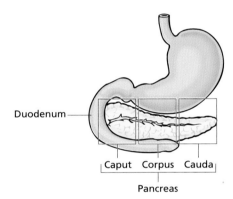

Figure 1.26 Position and gross anatomy of the pancreas.

The pancreas has two ducts that empty into the duodenum. Usually the main pancreatic duct empties together with the common bile duct at the papilla Vater.

Pancreatic secretion, like gastric secretion, is regulated by both nervous and hormonal mechanisms; however, the hormonal mechanisms are by far the most important of the two.

2 Swallowing Disorders

Dysphagia is used to describe the sensation of difficulty in swallowing, regardless of the cause or the localization of the problem.

Problems that can cause dysphagia are:

- disturbed swallowing reflex
- mechanical obstruction
- motility disorders
- gastroesophageal reflux disease (GERD).

2.1 Physiology

The mouth, tongue, pharynx, and the esophagus are the anatomic structures that are involved in swallowing.

The swallowing process can be divided into three separate stages (Figs 2.1 & 2.2):

1 voluntary or oral stage
2 pharyngeal stage
3 esophageal stage.

1 VOLUNTARY OR ORAL STAGE

Food on the tongue is voluntarily moved to the back of the mouth. The tongue forces the food into the pharynx.

2 PHARYNGEAL STAGE

Food is transported from the pharynx into the esophagus. This is a reflex action. The food stimulates swallow receptors in the pharynx sending impulses to the swallow center in the brainstem. This center inhibits respiration during this stage of the swallow and initiates a series of coordinated events to:

- prevent reflux of food to the nasal cavities
- prevent food from passing into the trachea
- widen the opening of the esophagus and relax the upper esophageal sphincter (UES)
- produce peristaltic waves that move the food down into the esophagus.

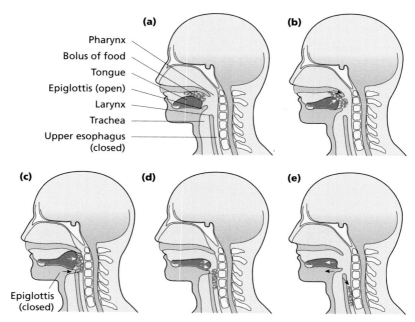

(a)
Pharynx
Bolus of food
Tongue
Epiglottis (open)
Larynx
Trachea
Upper esophagus
(closed)

(b)

(c)
Epiglottis
(closed)

(d)

(e)

Figure 2.1 Schematic representation of the movement of a bolus from the mouth to the upper esophagus during swallowing.

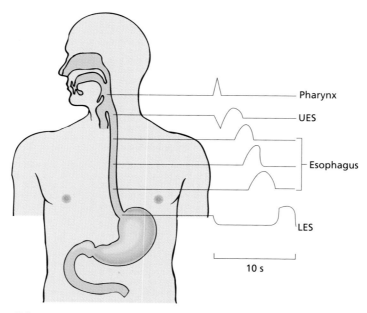

Pharynx

UES

Esophagus

LES

10 s

Figure 2.2 Manometric representation of normal swallowing movements.

3 ESOPHAGEAL STAGE

The food bolus is transported by gravity and peristalsis along the esophagus. Normally, it takes about 7–10 s for the food bolus to pass the entire 25-cm-long esophagus. The lower esophageal sphincter (LES) relaxes to allow food to pass into the stomach.

The LES normally has a resting pressure which is approximately 20 mmHg higher than the intragastric pressure. On swallowing, LES pressure decreases to approximately the same level as gastric pressure. The LES muscle opens allowing the bolus to pass down into the stomach. The sphincter does not close until the contraction has passed through.

LES resting pressure can vary depending on hormonal effects, medications, and the ingestion of different foods.

Factors that decrease LES pressure
- Hormones such as progesterone, secretin, cholecystokinin, and glucagon.
- Foods such as fat, alcohol, and chocolate.
- Medications such as calcium channel blockers, benzodiazepines, theophylline, and atropine.

Factors that increase LES pressure
- Hormones such as gastrin, motilin, and vasopressin.
- Food such as protein.
- Medications such as prokinetic drugs.

PERISTALSIS

In order to transport food to the stomach, there are two types of peristaltic contractions (Fig. 2.3).

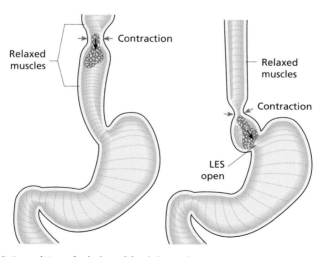

Figure 2.3 Propulsion of a bolus of food down the esophagus.

Primary peristalsis

Primary peristalsis is initiated by a swallow. The circular muscle layer contracts around the top of the food bolus and moves the food toward the stomach. The longitudinal muscle fibers below the bolus contract, shortening the esophagus and the passageway for the bolus.

Secondary peristalsis

Secondary peristalsis is initiated by the distention of the esophagus caused by retained material (food or refluxed material). This is of great importance for removing food from the esophagus if it has not been cleared totally by primary peristalsis. The initiation of this process continues until all remaining food has been cleared from the esophagus.

2.2 Oropharyngeal swallowing disorders

Structural or propulsive abnormalities of the oropharynx and/or the UES can disturb the normal swallowing process in different ways. Most cases of oropharyngeal dysfunction are the result of neurologic or muscular diseases and give rise to symptoms such as difficulty in controlling the food bolus within the oral cavity and initiating the pharyngeal swallow response. This leads to dysphagia for solid and liquid foods and difficulty in its passage from the mouth to the esophagus. The nasopharynx and airway may not be protected and serious respiratory consequences may arise.

Etiology

The causes of oropharyngeal swallowing disorders are:
- neuromuscular diseases which include congenital and acquired diseases of the central and peripheral nervous system such as cerebrovascular accidents, multiple sclerosis, Parkinson's disease, brainstem tumors, pseudobulbar palsy, peripheral neuropathy and muscular diseases (myasthenia gravis, poliomyelitis, dermatomyositis)
- mechanical obstruction such as compression from thyromegaly, cervical lymphadenopathy, oropharyngeal carcinomas, congenital abnormalities, inflammatory disorders, hyperostosis of the cervical spine
- iatrogenic defects caused by surgical dissection in the oropharyngeal area, radiotherapy, or as a result of operative or traumatic damage to the cranial nerves innervating the oropharynx.

Symptoms
- Oropharyngeal dysphagia (Fig. 2.4) for liquids and solid foods
- Oropharyngeal dysphagia with primarily difficulty in initiating the pharyngeal swallow response—often associated with speech difficulties, tongue paresis, and aspiration (common in swallowing disorders due to neuromuscular diseases)
- Nasopharyngeal regurgitation.

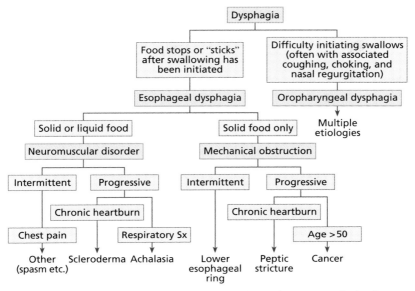

Figure 2.4 Algorithm for diagnosis symptom analysis of patients with dysphagia. Reproduced from Castell, 1992 with permission from Little Brown & Co.

Differential diagnosis
- Achalasia (symptoms may be falsely localized to UES)
- GERD
- Zenker's diverticulum (may be a consequence of UES dysfunction).

Diagnostic procedures
MORPHOLOGIC DIAGNOSTICS
Radiography with barium swallow
To visualize the swallowing process and to identify any obstructions.

Videoradiography
To evaluate oropharyngeal bolus transport, pharyngeal contraction, relaxation of the UES, and the dynamics of airway protection during barium swallowing. This is still the test of choice in the diagnostic evaluation of oropharyngeal swallowing disorders.

Endoscopy
To further evaluate obstructions, and to identify inflammation or neoplasm.

Videoendoscopic analysis
With a flexible laryngoscope the anatomic structures are visualized while swallowing. The closure of the nasopharynx and apposition of the vocal

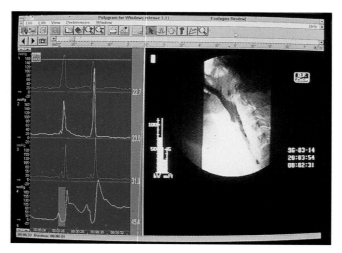

Figure 2.5 Synchronized barium swallow video manometry (from Medtronic GastroIntestinal).

cords are especially studied. The technique is also useful for detecting aspiration.

FUNCTIONAL DIAGNOSTICS

Pharyngeal manometry

In patients with dysphagia, where barium swallow studies prove normal or inconclusive, manometry can be useful. By performing manometry with specially designed catheters, it is possible to evaluate the swallowing process by determining the UES resting pressure, the relaxation of the UES, the pharyngeal contraction, and peristalsis. The coordination between UES relaxation and pharyngeal contraction is of particular interest (see Section 8.6).

Synchronized barium swallow video manometry (Fig. 2.5)

It is possible to combine pharyngeal manometry with simultaneous video-radiography in the evaluation of swallowing disorders. The video imaging and physiologic recordings are synchronized, displayed, and digitally recorded all on one computer.

Videoradiography

Demonstrates bolus transport through the pharynx and can identify its possible penetration into the airway. When combined with manometry, which records intraluminal pressure change, a detailed analysis of the pathogenesis of pharyngeal dysfunction is possible, which could not be obtained by either of these methods alone.

2.3 Zenker's diverticulum

Zenker's diverticulum is a hernia of the hypopharyngeal mucosa, located at the border between the pharynx and the esophagus. The diverticulum penetrates dorsally between the circular and oblique part of the cricopharyngeus muscle. When the patient swallows, food can easily be diverted into the hernia rather than down into the esophagus.

This leads to symptoms of dysphagia and delayed regurgitation of undigested food from Zenker's diverticulum.

Etiology

The etiology is not totally clear, but anatomic factors are of importance for the development of the diverticula. Also motor disorders of the UES and upper esophagus seem to be possible factors promoting the development of Zenker's diverticulum.

Two principal hypotheses have been proposed for the development of Zenker's diverticulum:
1 lack of coordination between UES relaxation and pharyngeal contraction
2 impaired opening of UES due to fibrosis or degeneration of its muscle fibers.

Symptoms
- Regurgitation of undigested food
- Dysphagia
- Appearance of a mass in the neck, especially after meals.

Differential diagnosis
- Oropharyngeal swallowing disorders
- Esophageal stricture
- Neoplasia.

Diagnostic procedures

Esophageal radiography with barium swallow
Radiography is the test of choice to visualize Zenker's diverticulum (Fig. 2.6).

Endoscopy
Endoscopy can also be used to visualize the diverticulum. However, there is a potential risk of perforating the thin mucosa of the diverticulum since it may be difficult to avoid entering the diverticulum.

Manometry
Pharyngeal manometry can define the coordination between pharyngeal peristalsis, UES relaxation and closure, and upper esophageal peristalsis. Manometry is useful preoperatively if surgery such as cricopharyngeal myotomy should be undertaken with diverticulectomy or diverticulopexy (see Section 8.6).

33

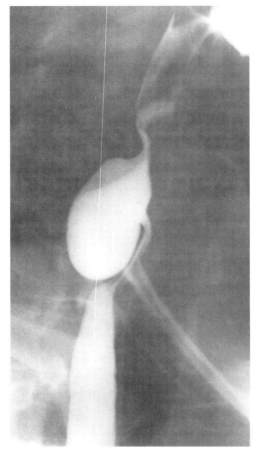

Figure 2.6 X-ray of Zenker's diverticulum. The pouch is lying behind the esophagus which is displaced forward.

2.4 Esophageal motility disorders

Esophageal motility disorders are often referred to as either primary, secondary, or nonspecific.

1 Primary esophageal motility disorders affect only one organ—the esophagus. Achalasia, diffuse esophageal spasm, and the nutcracker esophagus are all primary esophageal motility disorders

2 Secondary esophageal motility disorders reflect esophageal involvement by systemic diseases that affect many different organs. An example of a systemic disease which may cause an esophageal motility disorders is scleroderma

3 Nonspecific esophageal motility disorders may be associated with symptoms such as dysphagia or chest pain, but the abnormal pattern does not meet the criteria of a classical primary esophageal motility disorder.

1 Primary esophageal motility disorders
(a) Achalasia

Idiopathic achalasia is a primary esophageal motility disorder which gives rise to progressive dysphagia and regurgitation. The LES is usually hypertensive and, of greatest importance, does not relax completely on swallowing to let food pass into the stomach. Also, there is absence of distal esophageal peristalsis which leads to stasis of food and dilatation of the esophagus.

Etiology

The cause of achalasia has not been completely defined. Some data suggest an autoimmune process targeted at the nerves of the myenteric plexus, other evidence supports a genetic predisposition. Other data implicate infectious and environmental agents. The most consistent finding is the absence of inhibitory neurotransmitters (vasoactive intestinal peptide (VIP) and/or nitric oxide) at the LES which leads to the impaired relaxation.

Other abnormalities that have been observed in achalasia patients include:
- loss of ganglion cells within the myenteric plexus of the esophagus
- degenerative changes in the vagus nerve
- quantitative and qualitative changes of nerve cells in the dorsal motor nucleus of the vagus.

The net result is the combination of markedly impaired muscle activity in the esophagus (aperistalsis) and the unopposed contraction (instead of relaxation) of the LES on swallowing.

CHAGAS' DISEASE (SOUTH AMERICAN TRYPANOSOMIASIS)

This is a form of secondary achalasia. It results from a parasitic infection that destroys the ganglion cells of the myenteric plexus. This destruction leads to megaesophagus. Other organs of the gastrointestinal tract may also be affected.

Symptoms
- Dysphagia
- Regurgitation
- Substernal pain
- Aspiration
- Weight loss.

Differential diagnosis
- GERD with complications such as esophageal stricture
- Esophageal spasm
- Secondary motility disorders—scleroderma with associated peptic stricture
- Carcinoma (an achalasia-like syndrome has been described in relation to a number of tumors, most commonly carcinoma of the cardia).

35

If the patient is older at the onset of the symptoms, has a shorter duration of symptoms, modest dilatation of the esophagus, and rapid and profound weight loss, the likelihood of pseudoachalasia due to carcinoma increases.

Diagnostic procedures
MORPHOLOGIC DIAGNOSTICS
Esophageal radiography
Barium swallow X-ray is used to visualize the esophagus and demonstrate any esophageal dilatation. The characteristic X-ray appearance of achalasia is a dilated intrathoracic esophagus with an air–fluid level. The LES tapers to a point giving the esophagus a beak-like appearance (Fig. 2.7)

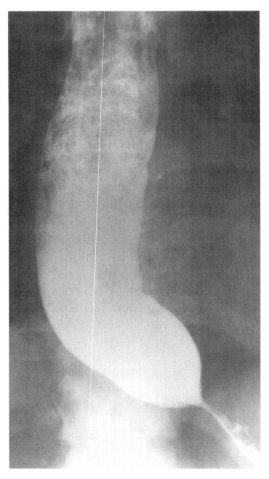

Figure 2.7 Radiography of the esophagus in a patient with achalasia.

Endoscopy

To rule out obstruction, esophagitis, or stricture, and to obtain biopsies to exclude neoplasm, etc.

FUNCTIONAL DIAGNOSTICS

Esophageal manometry (see Section 8.4)

The following are the characteristic manometric findings in achalasia (Fig. 2.8):

- absence of esophageal peristalsis
- elevated LES pressure (over 30 mmHg)
- absent, incomplete or complete but shortened (< 6 s) relaxation of the LES
- elevated intraesophageal pressure.

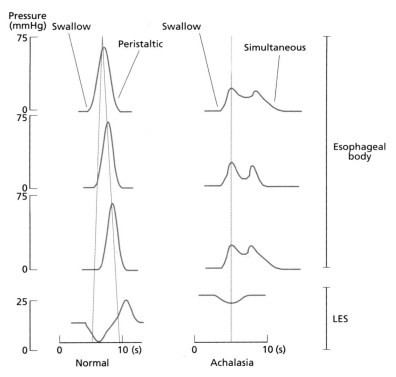

Figure 2.8 Schematic representation of manometric profile in a patient with achalasia. Reproduced from Smout, 1992 with permission from Wrightson Biomedical Publishing Ltd.

(b) Diffuse esophageal spasm

Diffuse esophageal spasm (DES) is a primary motility disorder of the esophagus. The patient presents with nonprogressive intermittent dysphagia that is often associated with chest pain. During manometry one sees simultaneous distal esophageal contractions mixed with normal peristalsis. True symptomatic DES is a rare condition.

Etiology

The etiology and neuromuscular pathophysiology of DES is still unclear.

Symptoms

- Substernal chest pain. The pain may also radiate to neck, arms, or jaw and may be associated with meals
- Intermittent dysphagia. Could be precipitated by stress, hot or cold liquids, or rapid eating
- Odynophagia (painful swallowing).

Differential diagnosis

- Ischemic heart diseases (IHD)
- GERD with complications such as esophagitis, stricture
- Achalasia
- Secondary motility disorders—scleroderma with associated peptic stricture
- Neoplasia.

Diagnostic procedures

MORPHOLOGIC DIAGNOSTICS

Endoscopy

To visualize the esophagus and rule out other conditions.

Esophageal X-ray with barium swallowing

In DES, it may reveal simultaneous nonperistaltic contractions with resulting segmentation of the barium column. This pattern is called the "corkscrew esophagus" (Fig. 2.9). Barium swallow is also used to rule out other conditions.

FUNCTIONAL DIAGNOSTICS

Esophageal manometry

The diagnosis of DES is based on the combination of appropriate clinical symptoms and certain manometric abnormalities (Fig. 2.10). On manometry, the specific manometric abnormalities which support the diagnosis of DES are:

- frequent simultaneous (nonperistaltic) contractions (more than 20–30% of wet swallows), separated by periods of normal peristalsis
- manometric abnormalities in DES are usually confined to the distal two-thirds of the esophagus
- multiphasic waves (more than two peaks per wave)
- prolonged duration of contractions (more than 6 s)
- spontaneous contractions
- high amplitude contractions (greater than 180 mmHg).

The last five points are common findings in patients with DES, but not necessary for the diagnosis of DES (see Section 8.4).

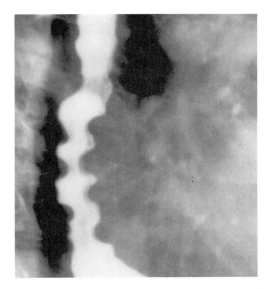

Figure 2.9 Corkscrew esophagus on barium X-ray in a patient with DES.

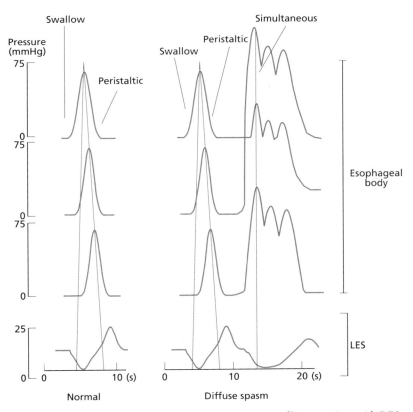

Figure 2.10 Schematic representation of the manometric profile in a patient with DES. Reproduced from Smout, 1992 with permission from Wrightson Biomedical Publishing Ltd.

(c) Nutcracker esophagus

The nutcracker esophagus is the most common manometric abnormality seen in patients with noncardiac chest pain (NCCP). Nutcracker refers to the combination of the esophageal manometric findings of high amplitude but peristaltic contraction waves in patients with chest pain or dysphagia.

Etiology

The etiology is unknown. Some dispute the existence of this condition as a real entity while others have speculated that the nutcracker can later progress to achalasia. An association with acid reflux and to stress have also been suggested.

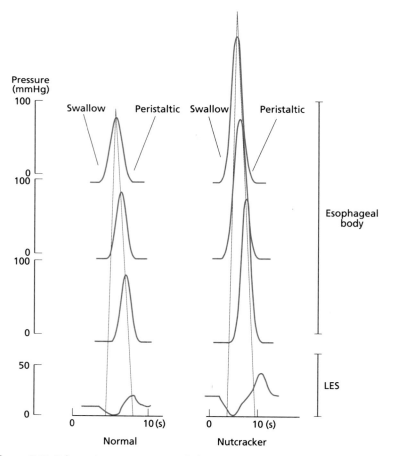

Figure 2.11 Schematic representation of the manometric profile in a patient with nutcracker esophagus. Reproduced from Smout, 1992 with permission from Wrightson Biomedical Publishing Ltd.

Symptoms
- NCCP
- Dysphagia (not as common as NCCP).

Differential diagnosis
- GERD
- IHD
- Achalasia
- DES
- Anxiety state.

Diagnostic procedures
FUNCTIONAL DIAGNOSTICS
Esophageal manometry

The following are manometric findings in Nutcracker esophagus (Fig. 2.11) (see Section 8.4):
- high amplitude peristaltic contractions typically above 180 mmHg. Contraction amplitudes can often exceed 300 mmHg
- prolonged duration contractions and elevated LES pressures are also seen but are not necessary for diagnosis.

2 Secondary motility disorders

Systemic diseases are diseases that can affect many different parts and organs of the body. Some of the systemic diseases (like scleroderma) can manifest in the esophagus and give rise to various degrees of dysfunction in this region, or in other words, secondary motility disorders.

(a) Scleroderma or progressive systemic sclerosis

Scleroderma is a disorder of the connective tissue which leads to fibrosis in multiple organs such as the skin, lungs, heart, GI tract, and the kidneys.

Etiology

The exact pathogenesis of the esophageal dysfunction is not clear. There is a predilection for the sclerodermatous changes to affect the smooth muscle in the distal two-thirds of the esophagus. The proximal part of the esophagus where striated muscle ocurs is not usually affected.

The fibrosis of the smooth muscle leads to diminished amplitude of peristalsis in the distal esophagus. In addition, incompetence of the LES occurs which can lead to severe gastroesophageal reflux and its complications such as:
- erosive esophagitis
- stricture
- Barrett's esophagus
- aspiration pneumonia.

41

Symptoms

- Heartburn
- Dysphagia
- Chest pain.

Differential diagnosis

- GERD
- Achalasia.

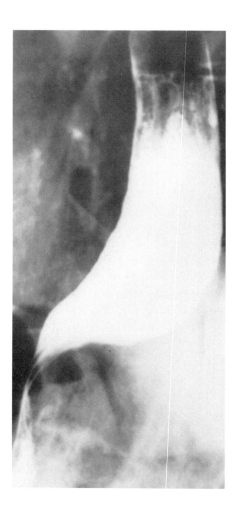
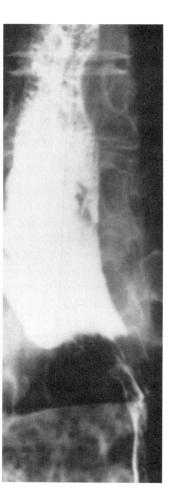

Figure 2.12 Barium swallow in a patient with scleroderma. On radiography, scleroderma can look similar to achalasia except for the wide open LES.

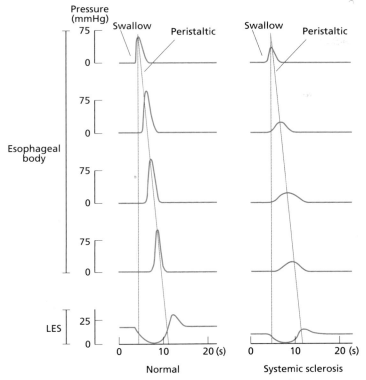

Figure 2.13 Schematic representation of the manometric profile in a patient with scleroderma. Reproduced from Smout, 1992 with permission from Wrightson Biomedical Publishing Ltd.

Diagnostic procedures

MORPHOLOGIC DIAGNOSTICS

Endoscopy

To evaluate for the presence of esophagitis or strictures. May obtain biopsies to exclude complications from gastroesophageal reflux such as esophagitis, Barrett's esophagus, etc.

Esophageal radiography with barium swallow

Esophageal body may variably appear dilated, atonic, or normal in diameter with diminished peristalsis (Fig. 2.12).

FUNCTIONAL DIAGNOSTICS

Esophageal manometry

With esophageal manometry one can find manometric abnormalities that suggests the diagnosis of scleroderma (see Section 8.4).

Manometric findings

- Decreased LES pressure (leading to gastroesophageal reflux)
- Weak or absent peristalsis in the distal esophagus
- Normal upper esophageal peristalsis and UES pressure (Fig. 2.13).

Radionuclide esophageal scintigraphy

The decrease in emptying of the esophagus is proportional to the loss of distal esophageal muscle tone.

3 Nonspecific esophageal motility disorders

A clear distinction between the nonspecific esophageal motility disorder and the classical primary esophageal motility disorders (such as achalasia, diffuse esophageal spasm, and nutcracker esophagus) is often not possible.

Many patients with symptoms of dysphagia or NCCP demonstrate a variety of esophageal contraction patterns on manometry that are not within the normal range yet do not meet the criteria of a classical primary motility disorder. These motility disorders are therefore called nonspecific esophageal motility disorders.

Etiology

This is unknown. In some cases the motor abnormality may be induced by the irritation of refluxed gastric juice. However, this is not always true since it can also be a primary event unrelated to the presence of reflux.

Symptoms

- NCCP
- Dysphagia.

Differential diagnosis

- DES
- Achalasia
- IHD

Diagnostic procedures

FUNCTIONAL DIAGNOSTICS

Esophageal manometry

With manometry one can find manometric abnormalities that suggest the diagnosis of nonspecific esophageal motility disorder (see Section 8.4). Each of these manometric findings may be included under the term nonspecific esophageal motility disorder:

- increased number of multipeaked or repetitive contractions
- contractions of prolonged duration
- nontransmitted contractions—interruption of peristaltic waves at various levels of the esophagus

- contractions of low amplitude (less than 12 mmHg in upper, less than 25 mmHg in mid and lower esophagus)
- isolated, abnormal, LES function.

3 Reflux Disorders

3.1 Gastroesophageal reflux

Gastroesophageal reflux is the retrograde movement of gastric contents through the lower esophageal sphincter (LES) to the esophagus. It is a common, normal phenomenon which may occur with or without accompanying symptoms.

The stomach normally secretes acid at a pH of 1.5–2.0; this contrasts with the luminal environment of the esophagus where pH is almost neutral (pH 6.0–7.0). Distal esophageal pH will thus decrease dramatically when gastroesophageal reflux occurs.

Gastroesophageal reflux may be divided into two categories depending on whether it is normal physiologic reflux or pathologic reflux which occurs in gastroesophageal reflux disease (GERD).

PHYSIOLOGIC REFLUX
- Occurs mainly after meals
- Does not normally cause symptoms
- Short duration of reflux episodes
- Physiologic reflux is infrequent during sleep.

PATHOLOGIC REFLUX (Fig. 3.1)
- Frequent reflux episodes of longer duration
- Reflux episodes occurring during the day and/or night
- May produce symptoms and inflammation/mucosal injury of the esophagus.

Etiology
GERD originates from the pathological reflux of acid gastric contents. There are many factors which can contribute to the development of GERD:
1 Incompetent lower esophageal sphincter
2 Transient lower esophageal sphincter relaxation
3 Deficient or delayed esophageal acid clearance
4 Gastric abnormalities that increase physiologic reflux.

1 INCOMPETENT LOWER ESOPHAGEAL SPHINCTER
Many patients with GERD have a mechanically incompetent LES. In such

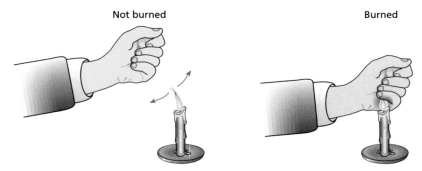

Figure 3.1 Pathologic reflux may produce symptoms and damage to the esophageal mucosa due to the extended acid exposure of the mucosa. The effects of acid reflux in the esophagus are analogous to the exposure of a hand to a candle flame. If the hand moves rapidly across the flame it will not get burned. If the hand stays too long over the flame, it will get burned.

cases if the intraabdominal pressure suddenly rises, reflux of gastric contents into the esophagus will occur.

The resistance to gastroesophageal reflux provided by the LES depends on several factors:

- LES pressure
- abdominal exposure of the LES
- overall LES length.

LES pressure

The LES has a higher basal or resting pressure than either the esophagus above and/or the stomach below. Normal pressure in the LES is 10–35 mmHg. The pressure varies with breathing, body position, body movements, and the migrating motor complex. There are also significant diurnal variations in LES tone with LES pressure being greatest during sleep and lowest following meals.

Low resting pressure in the LES is common among patients with severe reflux disease. The majority of GERD patients, however, have normal LES pressure, but the LES instead appears to be unusually prone to sudden transient lower esophageal sphincter relaxations (TLESRs) (see p. 50).

Table 3.1 Drugs that lower LES pressure.

Anticholinergic agents (or food with anticholinergic side effects)
Beta-adrenoceptor agonists (isoprenaline)
Theophylline
Benzodiazepines
Calcium blockers (verapamil, nifedipine)
Opiates

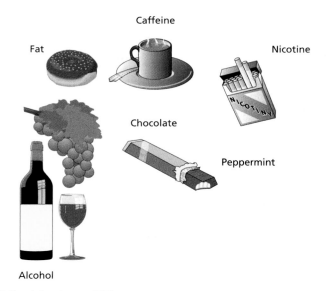

Figure 3.2 Food that lowers LES pressure.

Hormonal factors are also important to LES tone. During pregnancy, the increased levels of progesterone cause a decrease in the LES tone which together with the increased intraabdominal pressure and dislocation of the stomach can lead to problematic reflux.

Some drugs (Table 3.1) and even foods (Fig. 3.2) can decrease LES resting pressure and thereby cause increased reflux.

Length of LES exposed to the positive pressure environment of the abdomen
It is important that some part of the LES is located in the intraabdominal region where LES tone is augmented by exposure to intraabdominal pressure. When the pressure in the abdominal region increases, the LES is tightened (Fig. 3.3).

The lesser the intraabdominal length of the LES, the greater the risk of LES incompetency.

Overall LES length
The total length of the sphincter (normally between 2 and 5 cm) is also important in preventing reflux. The shorter the LES, the greater the likelihood of LES incompetence.

Hiatal hernias
LES function will be compromised by alterations in the anatomic relationships between the LES and the diaphragmatic crura (Fig. 3.4).

Contractions of the diaphragmatic crura serve to augment LES tone. During inspiration phasic crural contractions augment LES tone and protect

49

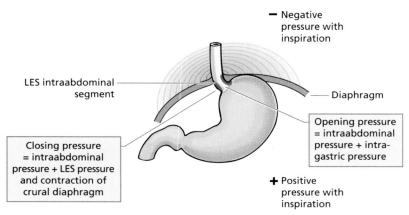

Figure 3.3 The LES and its location in the intraabdominal region. Closing and opening pressures at the LES.

against reflux at a time of elevated intraabdominal pressure. Otherwise the increase in abdominal pressure during inspiration would facilitate reflux.

In patients with a hiatal hernia the LES is displaced proximally and the diaphragm is now distal to the LES. During inspiration there is no increase in LES pressure since the contraction of the diaphragm occurs distal to the LES.

In the presence of a hiatal hernia the crural contractions will compromise esophageal emptying and impair esophageal acid clearance (see Fig. 3.4).

2 TRANSIENT LES RELAXATION (Fig. 3.5)

TLESR refers to episodes of LES relaxation that occur unrelated to the swallowing procedure (pressure decreases to the gastric level and lasts at least 10 s).

The understanding and control of the transient relaxation is incomplete, but it seems to be the most important factor underlying both physiologic

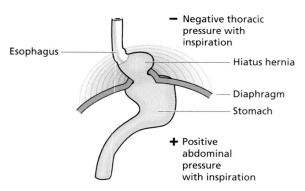

Figure 3.4 The effect of a hiatus hernia on esophagogastric junction anatomy.

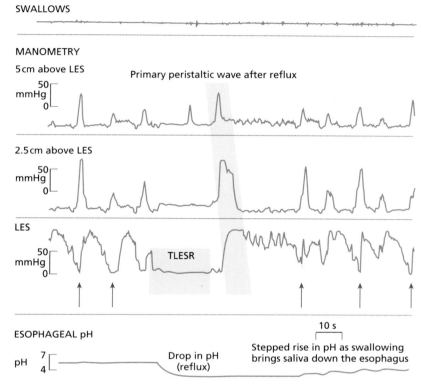

SWALLOWS

MANOMETRY

5 cm above LES

Primary peristaltic wave after reflux

2.5 cm above LES

LES

TLESR

10 s

ESOPHAGEAL pH

Stepped rise in pH as swallowing brings saliva down the esophagus

Drop in pH (reflux)

Figure 3.5 Manometric representation of a TLESR. The arrows point at LES relaxation during swallowing whereas the TLESR occurs unrelated to the swallowing procedure. There is a drop in pH during the TLESR. Reproduced with permission of The Medicine Group (Education) Ltd.

and pathologic gastroesophageal reflux. In GERD patients with normal LES pressure, TLESRs were found to be the most prevalent mechanism of reflux.

Gastric distention is thought to be one of the important triggering factors for TLESRs. The postprandial increase of both physiologic and pathologic gastroesophageal reflux may be due to this phenomenon.

3 DEFICIENT OR DELAYED ESOPHAGEAL ACID CLEARANCE

Three factors are important in esophageal clearance, which is defined as the return of esophageal pH to over 4.

1 Gravity
2 Esophageal motor activity:
   (a) Primary peristalsis—the pharyngeal swallow is initiated voluntarily and is the major esophageal motor activity that clears the esophagus of refluxed material. During the daytime a normal person swallows approximately 60 times per hour, initiating primary peristalsis with each swallow. At night the frequency of swallows is reduced to about six per hour

(b) Secondary peristalsis occurs in the absence of a pharyngeal swallow and can be elicited by esophageal distention or acidification; however, it infrequently results in the clearance of acid.

Esophageal peristaltic dysfunction results in ineffective clearance of acid from the esophagus and consequently prolonged esophageal acid exposure

3 Salivation results in the bicarbonate-rich natural buffer to acid in the esophagus. It neutralizes the minute amount of acid that is left after clearance by a peristaltic wave.

4 GASTRIC ABNORMALITIES THAT INCREASE PHYSIOLOGIC REFLUX

(a) Gastric dilatation and outlet obstruction

Outlet obstruction of the stomach

This may increase gastric pressure and/or gastric dilatation. This can result in reflux of gastric contents in the esophagus through a normal LES.

The outlet obstruction is often due to scarring and strictures of the gastric outlet caused by duodenal ulcers.

Vagotomy and diabetic neuropathy

These may cause increased gastric pressure since the normal receptive relaxation of the stomach is interrupted. The increased pressure may lead to reflux of gastric contents (Fig. 3.6).

Excessive gastric dilatation (Fig. 3.7)

As the stomach dilates, the LES sphincter becomes shorter which affects LES competence. Causes of excessive gastric dilatation are:

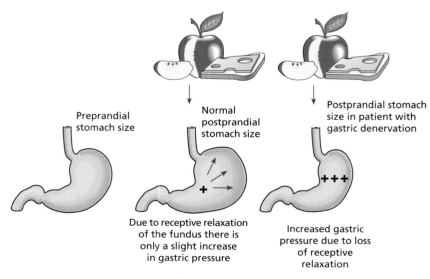

Preprandial stomach size

Normal postprandial stomach size

Postprandial stomach size in patient with gastric denervation

Due to receptive relaxation of the fundus there is only a slight increase in gastric pressure

Increased gastric pressure due to loss of receptive relaxation

Figure 3.6 Receptive relaxation is disrupted leading to increased gastric pressure.

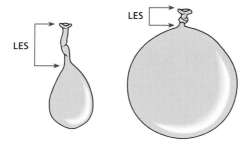

LES

LES

Figure 3.7 Stomach compared to a balloon. Excessive gastric dilatation leads to a shorter LES.

- aerophagia, in patients who reflux and habitually swallow to clear the esophagus
- overeating
- outlet obstruction of the stomach due to, for example, ulcer disease or malignancy.

(b) Delayed gastric emptying

A stomach, distended for prolonged periods, may facilitate the reflux of gastric contents during episodes of transient LES sphincter relaxations (TLESR). It has also been shown that gastric retention increases the frequency of transient relaxations.

Delayed gastric emptying can be caused by abnormalities such as:
- gastric atony from advanced diabetes
- diffuse neuromuscular disorders
- vagotomy
- idiopathic gastric paresis which may occur, for example, after viral infections
- pyloric dysfunction and duodenal dysmotility can also reduce gastric emptying.

A summary of the chief pathogenic factors involved in GERD is shown in Fig. 3.8.

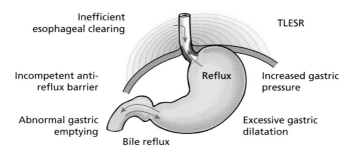

Inefficient esophageal clearing

TLESR

Incompetent anti-reflux barrier

Reflux

Increased gastric pressure

Abnormal gastric emptying

Excessive gastric dilatation

Bile reflux

Figure 3.8 Summary of chief pathogenic factors involved in GERD.

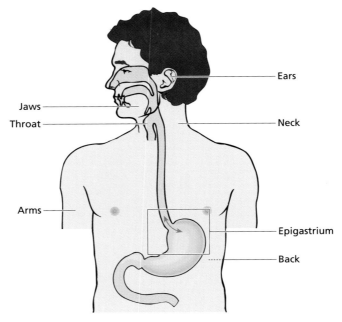

Figure 3.9 Possible distribution of pain in patients with GERD.

Symptoms

Symptoms associated with GERD include (Fig. 3.9):

- heartburn
- acid regurgitation
- chest pain
- dysphagia
- chronic cough
- hoarseness
- laryngitis
- asthma
- dental erosions.

GERD comprises a wide spectrum of pathological manifestations and may present with any one of a long list of diverse symptoms. Unfortunately, symptom severity is not an accurate predictor of disease severity. Furthermore, attempts to correlate reflux episodes with symptoms have shown that 85% of reflux episodes, defined as a drop in esophageal pH to less than 4, are asymptomatic.

Differential diagnosis

- Esophageal carcinoma
- Peptic ulcer

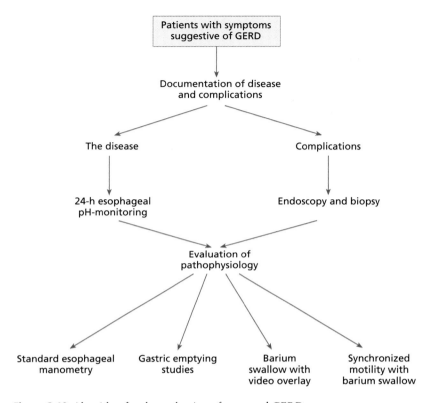

Figure 3.10 Algorithm for the evaluation of suspected GERD.

- Ischemic heart disease (IHD)
- Cholelithiasis
- Nonpeptic esophagitis.

Diagnostic procedures

The general scheme of investigating suspected GERD is shown in Fig. 3.10.

MORPHOLOGIC DIAGNOSTICS

Endoscopy and biopsy

- To assess macroscopic changes in the esophageal mucosa caused by gastroesophageal reflux. However, GERD may exist without any visible esophageal damage
- To exclude other pathological conditions that may cause the symptoms mentioned above.

Esophageal radiography with barium swallow

These are helpful in identifying GERD-related obstructive lesions such as rings and strictures; they can also provide a detailed assessment of esophageal and gastric anatomy as well as hiatal hernia size and location and also permit some assessment of esophageal propulsion (with barium swallow).

FUNCTIONAL DIAGNOSTICS

Gastroesophageal scintigraphy

A relatively simple noninvasive procedure. The patient is given a liquid or mixed liquid–solid meal labeled with a non-absorbable radioisotope, usually technetium. Transit of the labeled meal through the esophagus is then monitored by an external gamma counter.

However, the test's sensitivity and specificity in the diagnosis of GERD has been disputed. The conditions during the test are not physiological and observation is limited to a short period of time.

Esophageal manometry

Esophageal manometry is not diagnostic of GERD, but provides valuable information on pathophysiology. It measures LES pressure, position, and length, and the pattern of esophageal peristalsis. Esophageal manometry is also important to localize the LES for positioning of the pH electrode (see Section 8.4).

Ambulatory 24-h pH recording

This plays an important role in the documentation of pathological gastro-esophageal reflux (see Section 8.2). It provides a number of parameters:

- a quantitative measure of reflux duration
- information on reflux frequency
- information on when reflux occurs
- symptoms–reflux correlation
- information on the esophageal clearance of refluxed acid.

3.2 Duodenogastroesophageal reflux—bile reflux

Duodenogastroesophageal reflux means the reflux of duodenal contents, such as bile, pancreatic, and enteric juices to the stomach and esophagus.

Pathological reflux of duodenal contents to the stomach has been linked to the development of gastritis, gastric ulcers, gastric carcinoma, dyspepsia, and the postcholecystectomy syndrome. These associations remain, however, disputed and highly controversial.

Reflux of duodenal contents in the esophagus has been implicated, perhaps as a cofactor, with acid reflux, in the development of such complications of gastroesophageal reflux as esophagitis, Barrett's esophagus, and adenocarcinoma. Again, this is an area of considerable controversy and the role of bile reflux continues to be defined.

Etiology

While the pathophysiology of duodenogastric and duodenogastroesophageal reflux is far from clearly understood, several factors may be, in theory, at least relevant:

- sphincter incompetence: duodenal contents can easily reach the stomach and the esophagus through the pylorus and LES
- antroduodenal dysmotility—dyscoordination between the antrum, pylorus, and duodenum could lead to retrograde flow of duodenal contents
- post-hemigastrectomy—here the reflux barrier has been surgically removed (Fig. 3.11).

Duodenogastroesophageal reflux could exacerbate, in theory, gastroesophageal reflux in two ways:

- by increasing intragastric volume and thereby increasing the risk of gastroesophageal reflux
- by adding new components, such as duodenal juice with bile and pancreatic enzymes, that are potentially injurious to the mucosa of the esophagus.

Symptoms

Many individuals with documented duodenogastroesophageal reflux are asymptomatic. While the following symptoms have been linked with this type of reflux this association is far from well defined:

- regurgitation
- heartburn
- nausea
- abdominal distention
- bloating
- vomiting bile
- chest pain.

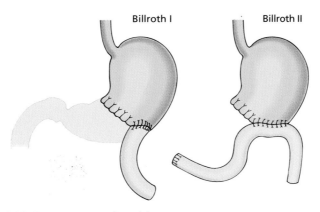

Figure 3.11 Common types of partial gastrectomy.

Differential diagnosis

- Acid gastroesophageal reflux
- Esophageal carcinoma
- Peptic ulcer
- Cholelithiasis.

Diagnostic procedures

MORPHOLOGIC DIAGNOSTICS

Endoscopy with biopsy

- To exclude other pathological conditions that may cause symptoms such as those listed above
- To document any damage of the esophageal or gastric mucosa that could be caused by duodenogastroesophageal reflux.

FUNCTIONAL DIAGNOSTICS

24-h pH monitoring

With combined 24-h esophageal and gastric pH monitoring, duodeno-gastroesophageal reflux can be suspected to a certain extent on the basis of elevation in intraesophageal pH, but it may be most difficult to identify mixed reflux episodes. Since duodenogastroesophageal reflux is often combined with acid reflux, esophageal pH may not rise when mixed reflux occurs. However, even if a pH rise is detected in the esophagus, it is also difficult to discriminate if the rise is due to duodenogastroesophageal reflux or related to the normal pH environment in the esophagus since saliva and many ingested foods have a pH > 7.

Ambulatory spectrophotometry

Refluxed duodenal contents contain bile which contains the pigment bilirubin. It is possible to detect bile reflux using bilirubin as a marker. On spectrophotometry bilirubin has a characteristic absorption peak at 453 nm, within the visible light spectrum (Fig. 3.12). Bilirubin can be

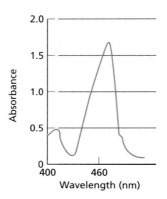

Figure 3.12 Absorption spectrum of bilirubin.

detected in the esophagus or stomach using a specific probe which carries light signals into the lumen of the gastrointestinal tract. The signals are then reflected back to an optoelectronic system in a fiberoptic bundle which then calculates the absorbance of the emitted light in the appropriate wavelength (453 nm)—absorption is proportional to the concentration of bilirubin in the lumen (see Section 8.3).

3.3 Manifestations of gastroesophageal reflux

1 Noncardiac chest pain

Noncardiac chest pain (NCCP) refers to chest pain that on clinical ground appears typical of pain of cardiac origin yet evaluation fails to identify cardiac disease. This pain may instead originate from the esophagus (Fig. 3.13).

Sensory nerve fibers from the esophagus follow the symphatic nerves to the spinal cord between T1 and T6; and predominantly between T4 and T6, an area that also receives sensory input from the heart.

This convergence of sensory fibers may explain why painful sensation from the esophagus may be confused with cardiac pain. This is commonly called referred pain.

However, pain receptors in the esophagus have not been clearly identified. Esophageal chest pain has been attributed to the stimulation of both chemo-receptors (acid and bile) and mechanoreceptors (spasm and distention). Also, the excitation of temperature receptors may cause chest pain of esophageal origin.

Etiology

Several factors have been proposed to explain chest pain of esophageal origin:
- abnormal esophageal acid exposure—50% of patients with NCCP have been found to have abnormal esophageal acid exposure
- motility abnormalities in the esophagus

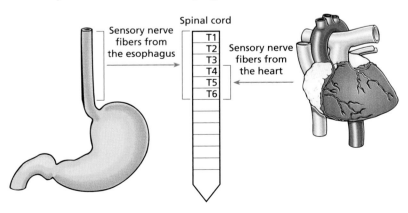

Figure 3.13 Sensory input from the esophagus and the heart.

- duodenogastroesophageal reflux exposure
- decreased sensory thresholds
- psychopathology.

Symptoms
Retrosternal chest pain.

Differential diagnosis
- IHD
- Pulmonary disorders
- Musculoskeletal pain.

Diagnostic procedures (Fig. 3.14)
MORPHOLOGIC DIAGNOSTICS
Endoscopy
Endoscopy with biopsy is used to exclude pathology such as esophagitis, esophageal ulcers, esophageal carcinoma, etc., as the cause of chest pain.

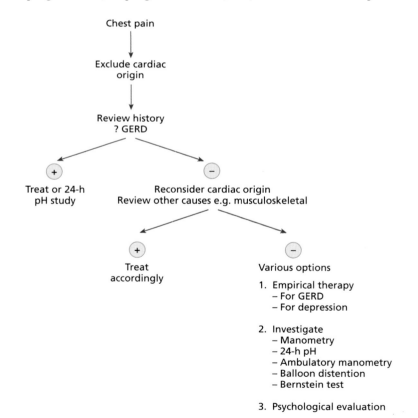

Chest pain

↓

Exclude cardiac origin

↓

Review history
? GERD

(+)
Treat or 24-h pH study

(−)
Reconsider cardiac origin
Review other causes e.g. musculoskeletal

(+)
Treat accordingly

(−)
Various options

1. Empirical therapy
   – For GERD
   – For depression

2. Investigate
   – Manometry
   – 24-h pH
   – Ambulatory manometry
   – Balloon distention
   – Bernstein test

3. Psychological evaluation

Figure 3.14 Algorithm for the evaluation of chest pain.

FUNCTIONAL DIAGNOSTICS
Acid perfusion test (Bernstein test)
Hydrochloric acid solution is perfused into the esophagus while the patient is in an upright or supine position. Alternating infusions of acid and saline are administered in a single blinded fashion, and the patient is instructed to report any symptoms. The test is considered positive if the patient's symptoms (such as chest pain) occur only during acid perfusion.

The use of this test has become less frequent due to the increased use of ambulatory esophageal pH-metry. Due to the relatively short observation period, the test is less sensitive than 24-h pH-metry.

24-h pH and manometry
Possible role includes:
- to determine if gastroesophageal reflux, abnormal esophageal motility, or other esophageal abnormalities may be the cause of chest pain once cardiopulmonary disorders has been conclusively excluded
- to correlate chest pain with abnormalities found on esophageal pH-metry or esophageal motility records.

By recording pH, motility, and electrocardiogram (ECG) events for 24 h, symptoms may be correlated with abnormalities in an attempt to prove that NCCP is of esophageal origin (see Section 8.5).

2 Esophagitis
Esophagitis refers to the inflammation of the mucosa of the esophagus.

Etiology
- Gastroesophageal reflux—the most common cause for esophagitis
- Duodenogastroesophageal reflux in an acid environment
- Accidental or suicidal ingestion of corrosive agents
- Fungal infections, especially *Candida albicans*, in debilitated or immuno-incompetent patients
- Viral—herpes simplex and cytomegalovirus, more frequent in the immuno-compromised
- Tuberculosis, syphilis (rare)
- Prolonged gastric intubation
- Uremia
- Dermatologic disorders such as pemphigus and epidermolysis bullosa
- Medications—"pill-esophagitis".

Symptoms
There is not a good correlation between symptoms and the endoscopic severity of esophagitis. Patients with severe symptoms may not necessarily have severe esophagitis.

chapter

3

Symptoms associated with esophagitis are therefore those related to GERD:

- heartburn
- retrosternal pain
- regurgitation/belching
- dysphagia/odynophagia
- asymptomatic.

Diagnostic procedure

ENDOSCOPY (Fig. 3.15)

This is the gold standard and permits both the visualization and classification of esophagitis and also permits biopsy of the esophageal mucosa.

The following is the Savary and Miller scheme for the endoscopic classification of esophagitis:

- Stage 1: one or more longitudinal non-confluent mucosal lesions with erythema, often covered with exudate above or extending from the gastroesophageal junction
- Stage 2: confluent erosive and exudative mucosal lesions which do not cover the entire circumference of the esophagus
- Stage 3: circumferential erosive and exudative lesions covering the whole esophageal mucous membrane
- Stage 4: chronic mucosal lesions such as ulcerations with or without stricture formation.

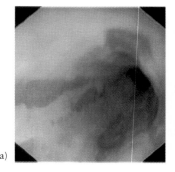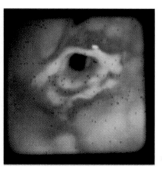

(a) (b)

Figure 3.15 Endoscopic views of the distal esophagus. (a) Linear hyperaemia with erosions: reflux esophagitis. Reproduced from Cotton & Williams, *Practical Gastrointestinal Endoscopy*, 3rd edn, 1990 (Blackwell Science, Oxford) with permission of the authors. (b) Peptic esophageal stricture.

Complications (Fig. 3.16)

- Stricture formation which may lead to dysphagia
- Ulceration which may lead to intensive pain radiating to the back, dysphagia, and hemorrhage.

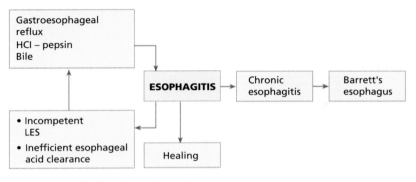

Figure 3.16 Pathophysiology of esophagitis.

3 Barrett's esophagus
Etiology
Barrett's esophagus is a complication of chronic GERD. The normal squamous epithelium of the distal esophagus has been replaced by metaplastic columnar epithelium in order to be more resistant to the damaging effect of refluxed juices (Fig. 3.17).

There are two important factors in the pathogenesis of Barrett's mucosa:
1 injury to the esophageal squamous epithelium
2 an abnormal esophageal environment as epithelial repair occurs.

These may in turn be related to:
• chronic reflux esophagitis
• duodenogastroesophageal reflux
• impaired acid clearance in conjunction with one of the factors above.

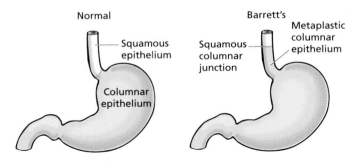

Figure 3.17 Barrett's esophagus.

Symptoms
Barrett's esophagus is a pathological condition which does not give rise to any symptoms in and of itself. Symptoms in patients with Barrett's

esophagus are related to the basic abnormality—GERD or its complications, such as ulceration and stricture.

Complications

The diagnosis of Barrett's esophagus is of major importance in view of its association with progression to adenocarcinoma of the esophagus.

The histological type of Barrett's esophagus is of key importance: intestinal metaplasia (recognized by the presence of goblet cells) is alone associated with progression to cancer in Barrett's esophagus.

Diagnostic procedure

ENDOSCOPY (Fig. 3.18) **WITH BIOPSY**

This is essential for the definition of Barrett's esophagus and for the identification of histological type, dysplasia and adenocarcinoma.

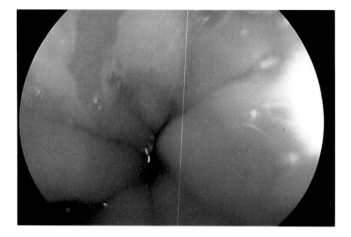

Figure 3.18 Endoscopy picture of Barrett's esophagus.

4 Pulmonary manifestations of gastroesophageal reflux

Gastroesophageal reflux is considered to be an important cause of chronic diseases of the larynx, the bronchial tree, and the lungs.

Asthma, chronic cough, bronchitis, aspiration pneumonia, laryngitis, and hoarseness can all be caused by reflux.

Etiology

The major defense against pulmonary aspiration of oral contents is the co-ordinated swallowing reflex which includes glottic closure and airway protection. The defenses against aspiration of refluxed gastric contents include the upper esophageal sphincter (UES) and the esophageal peristaltic

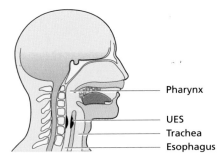

Pharynx

UES
Trachea
Esophagus

Figure 3.19 The UES prevents the reflux of gastric contents.

responses to refluxed material (Fig. 3.19). Coughing and bronchospasm defend the lungs once aspiration occurs. If some of these defense mechanisms are impaired, gastroesophageal reflux can cause pulmonary manifestations.

There are two possible mechanisms of gastroesophageal reflux related pulmonary disease:

- Injury related to actual aspiration of gastric contents. Refluxed material comes into direct contact with the bronchial surface which can lead to: (i) stimulation of the cough reflex; or (ii) mucosal damage resulting in bronchospasm or transudation of fluid into the airways
- Reflex response to reflux without actual aspiration. Asthma, coughing, or wheezing may be mediated through a reflex arc involving esophageal sensory receptors and an efferent pathway whose stimulation results in bronchospasm.

(a) Reflux-induced asthma

Many patients with nonallergic asthma have been shown to manifest abnormal gastroesophageal reflux on 24-h pH monitoring.

Especially in children, gastroesophageal reflux may be an important factor in the pathogenesis of asthmatic problems. Silent gastroesophageal reflux has been detected in many children with recurrent respiratory disorders.

Symptoms
- Wheezing
- Chronic cough
- Nocturnal asthma
- Hoarseness.

Indications for diagnostic procedure
- Patients with refractory asthma
- Unexplained chronic interstitial lung disease
- Recurrent pneumonia
- Chronic cough
- Hoarseness
- Recurrent laryngitis.

Diagnostic procedure
Dual channel 24-h pH-metry
To detect reflux into the proximal esophagus that may give rise to laryngitis and/or pulmonary problems, a dual channel 24-h pH-metry may be performed. One pH sensor should be located 5 cm above the LES and one sensor in the proximal esophagus (2–3 cm below the UES) (see Section 8.2).

(b) Reflux laryngitis
The larynx is extremely sensitive to acid. Laryngitis (inflammation of the larynx) may result from contact between the laryngeal mucosa and relatively minute amounts of acid.

Etiology
A substantial proportion of patients with voice abnormalities are believed to have chronic occult gastroesophageal reflux as an etiological factor.

Two theories have been proposed to explain the development of gastroesophageal reflux-related laryngitis:
- a vagally mediated reflex where the stimulus is acid in the lower esophagus and the response is chronic repetitive throat clearing and coughing which then lead to laryngeal lesions and symptoms
- direct acid injury to the larynx.

Symptoms
- Morning hoarseness
- Prolonged vocal warm-up
- Excessive phlegm
- Frequent throat clearing
- Dry mouth
- Coated tongue
- Chronic cough.

Indications for diagnostic procedure
- Presence of symptoms listed above
- If laryngeal examination shows laryngeal lesions such as erythema and edema suggestive of reflux-related injury.

Diagnostic procedures

MORPHOLOGIC DIAGNOSTICS

Laryngoscopy

- For direct visualization of laryngeal inflammatory changes that could be caused by reflux
- To exclude other pathological conditions that may cause similar symptoms.

Endoscopy

To visualize esophageal manifestations of GERD and if needed for taking biopsies from the esophageal mucosa.

FUNCTIONAL DIAGNOSTICS

Dual channel 24-h pH-metry (Fig. 3.20)

By using a two-channel electrode assembly, with one pH sensor located at 5 cm above the LES, and one sensor in the proximal esophagus (2–3 cm below the UES) it is possible to identify proximal acid reflux (see Section 8.2).

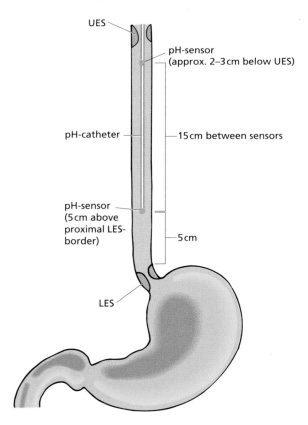

UES

pH-sensor
(approx. 2–3 cm below UES)

pH-catheter

15 cm between sensors

pH-sensor
(5 cm above
proximal LES-
border)

5 cm

LES

Figure 3.20 Location of pH sensors in the esophagus to detect high reflux.

4 Gastric and Small Intestinal Disorders

4.1 Physiology of the stomach and small intestine

Several clinical syndromes may be related to motor abnormalities of the stomach and proximal portions of the small bowel. The common symptom of indigestion, for example, may be a consequence of disturbed gastric motor function.

In the stomach, motility:
- mixes and grinds food
- regulates the emptying of gastric contents into the duodenum
- facilitates vomiting, when appropriate.

In the small intestine, motility:
- mixes the food with the digestive juices
- promotes contact between the products of digestion and the digestive–absorptive surface (the mucosa) of the small intestine
- propels waste products distally.

The fundus and the proximal part of the corpus of the stomach receive the ingested food and function as a reservoir.

The volume in the stomach can increase from approximately 300 to 1500 ml with barely a rise in intragastric pressure. This adaptive mechanism, receptive relaxation, which makes it possible to eat a huge meal quickly, is generated by a vagal reflex. This mechanism protects against the consequences of a sudden rise in intragastric pressure which could lead to the rapid emptying of gastric contents into the duodenum or, if the lower esophageal sphincter (LES) was incompetent, to the reflux of contents back into the esophagus (Fig. 4.1).

The mixing and grinding of food, and the emptying of gastric contents into the duodenum, are dependent on peristaltic contractions generated in the distal two-thirds of the stomach. These peristaltic contractions are controlled by the pacemaker of the stomach.

The pacemaker
The pacemaker area, which generates electrical impulses for gastric motility, is located on the greater curvature of the corpus of the stomach (Fig. 4.2).

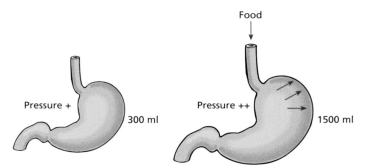

Figure 4.1 The receptive relaxation of the proximal part of the stomach accommodates the meal and prevents a sudden rise in intragastric pressure.

A wave of electrical depolarization, with a frequency of 3 cycles/min, radiates in a circumferential fashion through the stomach from the pacemaker area down toward the pylorus and the duodenum. This is called slow wave or electrical control activity (ECA) (Fig. 4.3).

However, when spike potentials are superimposed on slow waves, mechanical activity, such as a peristaltic contraction, is triggered. This may result from either hormonal or neural stimulation.

Consequently, since the slow wave mechanism normally has a frequency of 3/min in the stomach, the normal maximal contraction frequency is also 3/min in the stomach.

In the small intestine, the smooth muscle generates a cyclic change in membrane potential at a frequency of 10–12 cycles/min. When spike activity superimposes on this slow wave and depolarization reaches a critical threshold, contractions occur in the small bowel. The normal maximum contraction frequency is therefore 10–12/min in the small intestine (Fig. 4.4).

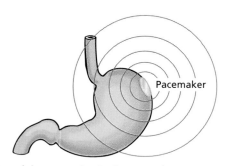

Figure 4.2 Location of the pacemaker in the stomach.

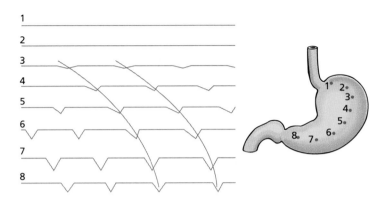

Figure 4.3 Electrical activity at various points in the stomach. Slow waves radiate from the pacemaker.

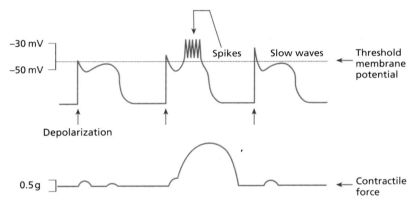

Figure 4.4 Smooth muscle contractions occur when spike activity superimposes on the slow wave and depolarization reaches a critical threshold. Reproduced with permission of The Medicine Group (Education) Ltd.

The migrating motor complex

Motor activity of the stomach and small intestine differs fundamentally depending on whether a person is fasting or has eaten recently.

FASTING

The migrating motor complex (MMC), which can be described as a band of motor events that starts in the stomach and travels distally through the small bowel, is the dominant pattern in the fasting state. The MMC can, however, also start at any place in the small intestine and travel distally from there.

The MMC is thought to have a clearance function. It protects the stomach and the small bowel from bacterial overgrowth in two ways:

71

1 it mechanically moves debris and bacteria distally
2 it lubricates (washes) the stomach and intestines since the MMC is associated with a cyclic increase in gastric acid secretion as well as bile and pancreatic juice flow.

The MMC returns some hours after the ingestion of food (how long depends on the caloric intake and the volume of the meal). The stomach feels empty, and hunger sensations begin.

During the day, the fasting period in between food intake is often short (less than 4 h), and consequently the MMC will often not be initiated. This is the main reason that the MMC occurs mainly during the night.

The MMC is composed of three distinct patterns of motor activity (Fig. 4.5):
- Phase 1: quiescence with no motor activity; lasts for 45–60 min. This phase is associated with absorption of fluid in the small bowel
- Phase 2: sporadic contractions that increase in amplitude and frequency over a 30–45 min period. This phase is associated with increased hydrochloric acid (HCl) secretion in the stomach and luminal flow in the small bowel
- Phase 3: the most distinct phase which features an uninterrupted band of regular contractions, which occur at the maximum rate of 3/min in the stomach and 10–12/min in the small bowel. This phase lasts for 2–12 min. These forceful contractions move the contents of the intestines distally.

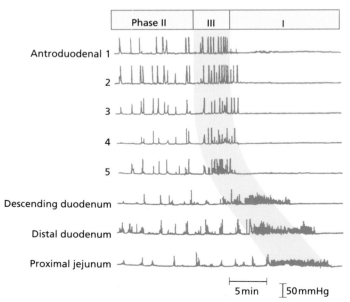

Figure 4.5 Normal fasting motor activity. Reproduced from Malagelada, 1986 with permission from Georg Thieme Verlag.

The enteric nervous system (plexus myentericus) is primarily responsible for the generation and propagation of the MMC. The hormonal control mediating phase 3 is accomplished mainly by the hormone motilin; however, many other hormones may also have a role in MMC modulation.

POSTPRANDIALLY

Immediately after the start of a meal, the MMC pattern is disrupted, and is replaced by a different pattern—the fed motor response. The stomach begins producing another form of contraction (Fig. 4.6).

Within a few minutes of the start of the meal, the stomach generates a stable pattern of intense peristaltic contractions. The contraction frequency approximates 3/min, and promotes optimal mixing and grinding of solid food.

There is a lag phase of 30–60 min after eating before the antral activity allows emptying of solids into the duodenum.

In the small intestine, food ingestion leads to the development of intense but irregular contractions that persist as long as there are nutrients in the lumen. The contractions are both segmental, to increase the contact of the food with the absorptive surface, and propulsive, to transport the content distally, usually over short segments.

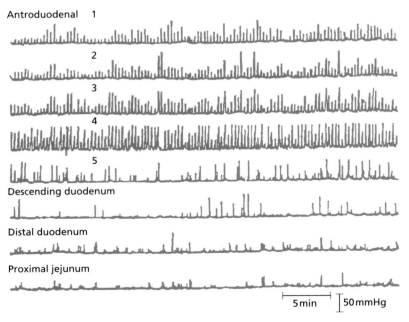

Figure 4.6 Normal fed (after a solid meal) motility reading. Reproduced from Malagelada, 1986 with permission from Georg Thieme Verlag.

4.2 Gastroparesis

Gastroparesis describes a motility disorder that results in delayed gastric emptying.

There is a huge range between extreme gastroparesis (gastrostasis, when there is no emptying of the stomach) and slightly delayed gastric emptying.

Etiology
See Table 4.1.

Symptoms
- Early satiety
- Epigastric burning or pain
- Bloating
- Nausea
- Vomiting, especially late postprandial
- Weight loss.

Differential diagnosis
- Gastroesophageal reflux
- Dyspepsia.

Table 4.1 Etiology of gastroparesis.

Mechanical obstruction	Scarring related to gastric or duodenal ulcers. Tumor
Endocrine/metabolic diseases	Diabetes with poor glycemic control or ketoacidosis. Diabetic neuropathy. Hypothyroidism. Electrolytes imbalance (K^+, Ca^{2+})
Postgastric surgery	Vagotomy. Partial gastrectomy. Outlet obstruction. Roux-en-Y syndrome
Systemic diseases	Scleroderma
Pseudoobstruction	Idiopathic. Secondary, for example, to muscular dystrophy
Central nervous system disease	Brainstem tumor. Raised intracranial pressure
Trauma	Head injuries. Burns. Spinal injury. Multiple trauma
Medication	Anticholinergics, opioids, L-dopa. Drug abuse (opiate narcotics)
Infections	Cytomegalovirus gastritis. Postviral gastroparesis
Idiopathic	May be related to underlying dysmotility, including tachygastria, antral hypomotility or gastroduodenal dyscoordination

Diagnostic procedures

Radiography

Barium studies can define mechanical obstructions, and may detect evidence of delayed gastric emptying. However, it is not possible to quantify gastric emptying accurately with this procedure.

Scintigraphy

Using a gamma camera it is possible to measure the emptying of a radio-labeled test meal containing solids and/or liquids. This is a noninvasive method which provides a reasonably precise quantification of gastric emptying. Changes in counts in the region of interest, detected by the gamma camera, reflect gastric emptying and can be monitored continuously to develop curves of gastric emptying.

However, the use of radioactive isotopes precludes this investigation during pregnancy and repeated studies in individual patients are, similarly, not recommended.

Absorption of orally administered drugs

After ingestion of a liquid meal containing paracetamol, for example, the concentration of paracetamol is measured in the blood. The absorption of paracetamol starts as soon as the paracetamol has been emptied into the duodenum. The concentration of paracetamol in the blood over time can therefore be used as an index of gastric emptying.

Ultrasound

After the ingestion of a liquid meal, the volume of the antrum is measured by ultrasound. The decrease of volume in the antrum correlates to the gastric emptying.

Electrical impedance

If a test meal has electrical conductivity that differs from the surrounding tissues, it is possible to measure the change in impedance across the abdominal wall using external electrodes. Changes in impedance correlate to the decrease of volume in the stomach during gastric emptying.

Breath test

By administering a test meal containing a small dose of ^{13}C octanoic acid, it is possible to trace the movement of solid food using breath analysis alone. When octanoic acid enters the duodenum, the tracer is rapidly absorbed and transported to the liver where it is oxidized. As a result, CO_2 is produced and exhaled where it can be detected in the breath. Postdose breath samples are collected at timed intervals and analyzed to provide an estimate of gastric emptying. ^{13}C is a stable isotope; radiation exposure is, therefore, not a concern.

In liquid food, ^{13}C sodium acetate is used as the radiolabel.

Ambulatory gamma counter

An isotope-sensitive, intragastric probe is placed in the stomach or the duodenum. The patient is then allowed to eat a radiolabeled meal and its elimination from the stomach can be continuously monitored to define delayed gastric emptying (see Section 8.9).

Electrogastrography

Electrogastrography (EGG) is a noninvasive technique that permits prolonged and repeated recordings of gastric electrical activity. By placing electrodes on the abdominal wall, above the stomach (Fig. 4.7), it is possible to record the electrical rhythm of the stomach which regulates peristalsis (Fig. 4.8). The relative amplitude and frequency changes of the EGG are associated with changes in gastric motility (see Section 8.8).

Disturbances of the EGG pattern have been described in many functional disturbances of the stomach (Fig. 4.9).

Since gastric myoelectrical activity is one of the factors that generate gastric emptying it should come as no surprise that EGG dysrhythmias are commonly documented in patients with proven gastroparesis.

It has been proposed that the EGG may serve as a screening tool for gastric dysmotility. Abnormalities in frequency and power response to a standardized meal are sensitive and specific indicators of gastric motor dysfunction (see Section 8.8).

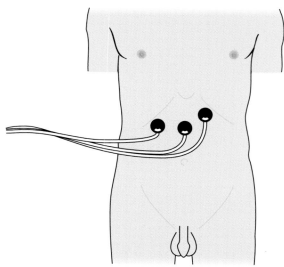

Figure 4.7 Location of surface electrodes for EGG recordings.

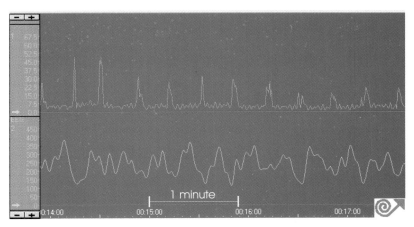

Figure 4.8 Simultaneous postprandial EGG and antral manometry showing regular 3 cycles/min slow waves on the EGG, which correspond to the manometrically measured phasic contractions at 3 cycles/min.

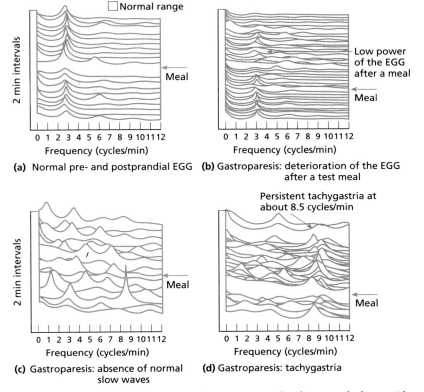

Figure 4.9 EGG used to differentiate between normal subjects and those with gastroparesis. Reproduced from Chen and McCallum, 1992 with permission from the *American Journal of Gastroenterology*.

4.3 Chronic dyspepsia

Chronic dyspepsia is a common clinical syndrome. Its definition is based on the presence of meal-related symptoms in the upper gastrointestinal tract when organic diseases have been excluded. Many patients with functional dyspepsia have been found to have motility abnormalities in the gastro-intestinal tract.

Functional dyspepsia may be classified into subgroups depending on the dominant symptom etiology:

- reflux-like symptoms
- ulcer-like symptoms
- dysmotility-like symptoms
- idiopathic, or unspecified functional dyspepsia.

The validity of this approach has been questioned, however, given the inconsistent relationship between symptom pattern and dysfunction.

Etiology

A number of mechanisms have been proposed to explain the pathogenesis of symptoms in dyspepsia.

- Gastrointestinal motor dysfunction including:

   (a) abnormal phasic contractile activity (esophagus, stomach, small bowel)

   (b) abnormal gut wall tonic activity in the basal state or in response to food, air, and fluid

   (c) delayed gastric emptying

- Mucosal infection/inflammation (gastritis, duodenitis)
- Hypersecretion of gastric acid
- Abnormal duodenogastric or gastroesophageal reflux
- Stress and psychosocial factors may play a role since they can alter intestinal secretion, motility, and blood flow
- Enhanced gastroduodenal sensitivity. Gastric volumes required to induce sensations of distention and pain are lower in patients with functional dyspepsia than in healthy people.

Symptoms

- Abdominal pain and/or discomfort with a duration of at least 1 month
- Postprandial fullness
- Early satiety or inability to finish a normal meal
- Bloating
- Nausea and/or vomiting
- Belching
- Heartburn
- Regurgitation
- Anorexia.

Differential diagnosis (Fig. 4.10)

- Peptic ulceration
- Gastritis caused by *Helicobacter pylori* infection
- Gastroesophageal reflux
- Gastrointestinal cancer
- Irritable bowel syndrome
- Cholelithiasis
- Chronic pancreatitis
- Gastroparesis
- Aerophagy.

Diagnostic procedures

Antroduodenal manometry (Fig. 4.11)

If investigations such as endoscopy, radiography, and pH recording, etc., have proven noncontributory, manometry may be considered to define dysmotility further (see Section 8.7).

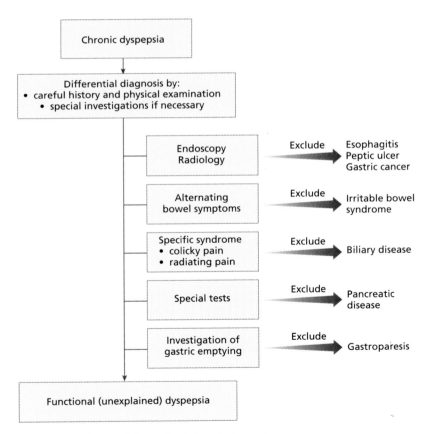

Figure 4.10 Differential diagnosis of chronic dyspepsia.

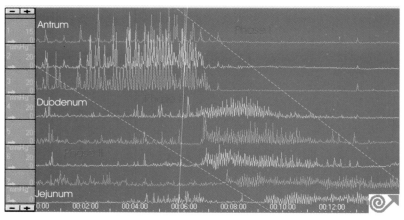

(a)

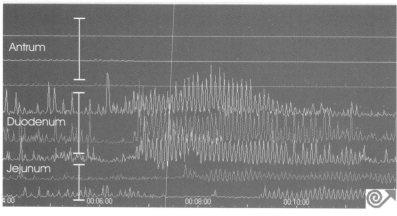

(b)

Figure 4.11 Antroduodenal manometry in the fasting state. (a) Normal patient shows phase III activity in antral channels. (b) Patient with dyspepsia shows that phase III activity of the migrating motor complex is absent in the antral channels.

Specific manometric patterns
- Postprandial hypomotility in the antrum—contraction frequency and amplitude are less in patients with dyspepsia compared to healthy people. This can lead to delayed gastric emptying which is also common in patients with functional dyspepsia
- Phase 3 of the MMC in the stomach is often missing in dyspepsia patients
- Duodenal motility disturbances are also common.

Electrogastrography
EGG can be used to detect gastric electrical dysrhythmias, which may be associated with symptoms of dyspepsia (see Section 8.8).

4.4 Chronic intestinal pseudoobstruction

Intestinal pseudoobstruction is a clinical syndrome defined by the presence of symptoms and signs of intestinal obstruction yet there is no evidence of mechanical blockage.

There are two principal clinical types of intestinal pseudoobstruction—chronic and acute pseudoobstruction (Fig. 4.12):

- Chronic intestinal pseudoobstruction (CIP) is a syndrome with a duration of months or years. The disease process may be relatively localized, or it may include the whole gastrointestinal tract from the esophagus to the rectum.

  The symptoms of intestinal obstruction are caused by the abnormal neuromuscular function of the small intestines and/or the colon, which results in ineffective intestinal propulsion

- CIP should be distinguished from acute intestinal pseudoobstruction, which is synonymous with acute ileus. Acute pseudoobstruction is often secondary to illnesses such as myocardial infarction, renal colic, or acute pancreatitis. Acute pseudoobstruction will typically resolve when the primary disease process is diagnosed and cured.

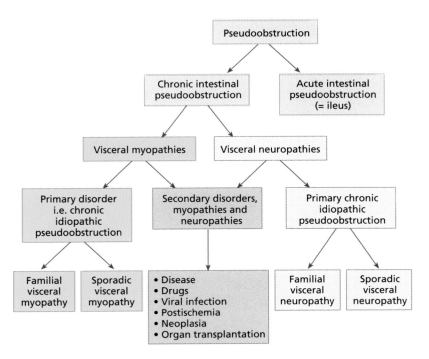

Figure 4.12 Pseudoobstruction.

Etiology

A variety of heterogeneous disease processes may result in the syndrome of CIP. Either the intestinal smooth muscle or the myenteric plexus in the gut are affected.

- Visceral myopathies reflect involvement of intestinal smooth muscle and may be accompanied by abnormalities of smooth muscle in other organs, such as the iris, the bladder, and the ureters
- Visceral neuropathies reflect abnormalities of the myenteric plexus, are more frequent than intestinal myopathies, and may be accompanied by abnormalities of the central, peripheral, or autonomic nervous system. CIP may therefore occur in association with mental retardation, Parkinsonism and autonomic nervous system dysfunction.

Both myopathies and neuropathies may be classified into two main groups:
1 Primary disorders (also called chronic idiopathic intestinal pseudo-obstruction (CIIP)), are most commonly congenital in origin and include:
  - familial visceral neuropathies and myopathies
  - sporadic visceral neuropathies and myopathies
2 Secondary disorders
  - CIP secondary to systemic diseases such as scleroderma, amyloidosis, myotonic dystrophy, diabetes mellitus, and hypothyroidism
  - CIP secondary to such drugs as tricyclic antidepressants, phenothiazines, L-dopa, antihypertensives (clonidine, ganglionic blockers), and laxatives
  - Following viral infections
  - Postischemic
  - Associated with multiple endocrine neoplasia
  - Paraneoplastic CIP.

Symptoms (Fig. 4.13)

Symptoms related to esophageal involvement
- Dysphagia or odynophagia
- Heartburn and other symptons of GERD.

Symptoms related to gastric and small intestinal involvement
- Abdominal pain
- Nausea
- Vomiting
- Bloating
- Distention and abdominal discomfort
- Malabsorption and malnutrition
- Diarrhea—due to bacterial overgrowth.

Symptoms related to colonic involvement
- Decreased passage of flatus
- Constipation

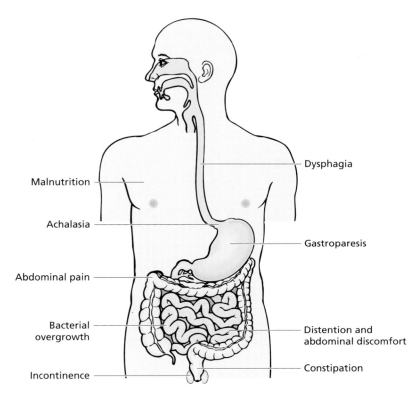

Malnutrition

Dysphagia

Achalasia

Gastroparesis

Abdominal pain

Bacterial overgrowth

Distention and abdominal discomfort

Incontinence

Constipation

Figure 4.13 Clinical findings. Pseudoobstruction may be localized, or can affect the entire gastrointestinal tract.

- Alternating diarrhea and constipation
- Incontinence.

Differential diagnosis
- Mechanical obstruction in the small bowel and/or colon
- Nonulcer dyspepsia
- Irritable bowel syndrome
- Chronic idiopathic constipation
- Gynecological disorders, e.g. endometriosis, pelvic inflammatory disease, ovarian carcinoma.

Diagnostic procedures
Radiography
Barium contrast studies of the entire gastrointestinal tract are of crucial importance in order to exclude mechanical obstructions. In pseudoobstruction, barium studies may also demonstrate delayed transit of barium which gives some indication of the extent of intestinal involvement.

4

chapter

83

The probability for CIP is greater if multiple parts of the gastrointestinal tract are involved.

On radiography myopathic forms of CIP may show:
- hypocontractility and dilatation of the small intestine and the colon
- loss of haustration in the colon.

In all types of CIP, the stomach may be enlarged and exhibit delayed emptying (gastroparesis) (see Section 4.2).

Transit studies
Radiolabeled meals can be followed through the small intestine and provide a quantifiable estimate of intestinal transit. In the colon transit can be estimated by radiographic assessment of the progress of radioopaque markers. Transit studies may help to measure the degree of stasis and to determine the severity of the disease.

Laparoscopy/laparotomy
The histopathologic diagnosis of an intestinal myopathy or neuropathy depends on the expert pathological examination of full-thickness samples of the intestinal wall, which can only be obtained either at laparotomy or laparoscopy. Some feel that these procedures should be avoided to reduce the risk of subsequent adhesion-related obstructions.

Esophageal manometry
The majority of patients with CIP exhibit abnormalities in esophageal peristalsis. The finding of abnormal peristalsis helps to support the diagnosis of CIP, but of course normal peristalsis does not exclude the disease. There are no specific esophageal manometric patterns suggesting CIP diagnosis (see Section 8.4).

Electrogastrography
This is not presently used in clinical practice but research suggests that this might be valuable as a noninvasive screening test for CIP among patients with suspected neuromuscular diseases of the gut. Persistent fasting tachygastria has been reported as highly suggestive of the neuropathic variety of pseudoobstruction (see Section 8.8).

Gastric and small bowel manometry
This is considered the most sensitive diagnostic tool for detecting CIP. It recognizes motor abnormalities even in mild cases prior to detection by radiographic, scintigraphic, or bowel transit studies (Fig. 4.14) (see Section 8.7).

Manometric findings
There are abnormalities of the motor patterns in both visceral myopathies and visceral neuropathies.

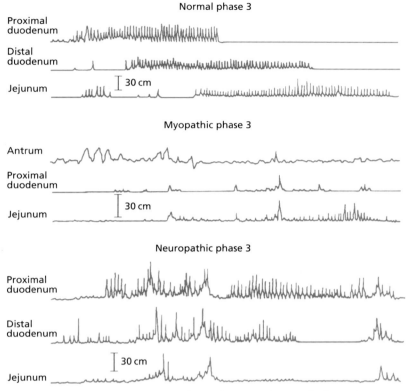

Figure 4.14 Phase 3 activity in myopathic and neuropathic pseudoobstruction compared to a healthy person. Reproduced from *Motilitet i ett kliniskt perspektiv* with permission from Janssen Cilag.

- *Visceral myopathies*: While the overall organization of the basic motor patterns (the MMC and the fed response) is preserved, the amplitude of individual phasic pressure waves is strikingly diminished.
- *Visceral neuropathies*: Individual pressure waves are of normal amplitude but their organization is disrupted.

Abnormal patterns described in neuropathic CIP include:
- abnormal configuration and propagation of the MMC
- uncoordinated bursts of phasic pressure activity
- uncoordinated intestinal pressure activity sustained for more than 30 min
- failure of a meal to induce a fed pattern.

A summary of the investigations which should be carried out when pseudo-obstruction is suspected is given in Fig. 4.15.

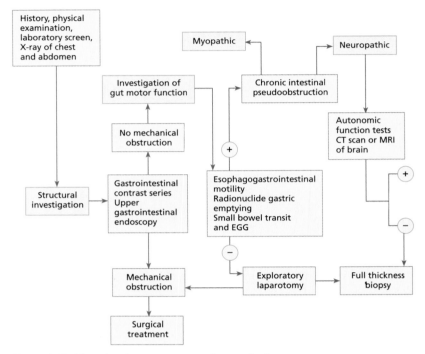

Figure 4.15 Algorithm for investigation of a pseudoobstruction.

4.5 Sphincter of Oddi dyskinesia (Fig. 4.16)

Obstruction of flow through the sphincter of Oddi may lead to biliary symptoms. If the patient shows such symptoms and abnormal sphincter of Oddi motility can be recorded, this is called sphincter of Oddi dyskinesia.

The obstruction may induce retention of bile and/or pancreatic juice in the common bile and pancreatic duct. This can lead to bile stasis and/or acute pancreatitis. The disturbed gallbladder emptying may also cause gallstones to

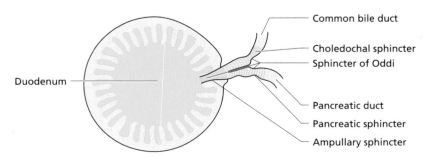

Figure 4.16 Anatomy of the sphincter of Oddi.

form. In other words gallstones are not always the primary cause of obstruction but may also be a consequence of flow obstruction of bile due to dyskinesia.

Sphincter of Oddi dyskinesia is common in patients with postcholecystectomy pain without demonstrable organic abnormality, its likelihood increases with increasing evidence of obstruction (increased level of enzyme values, delayed emptying, dilatation of bile duct, delayed contrast drainage).

Physiology

Alterations in sphincter of Oddi tone and phasic activity regulates the entry of bile into the duodenum (Fig. 4.17).

After a meal (especially a fat meal) there is a requirement of bile in the duodenum for absorption of fatty substances. The gallbladder muscle contracts and the sphincter of Oddi opens so that bile can flow easily to the duodenum.

In the fasting state the activity of the sphincter of Oddi is more complex. There is a tonic contraction of the sphincter of Oddi allowing it to be constricted much of the time, but also phasic contractions that are generally propagated toward the duodenum. This helps to keep the common bile duct dry by milking the bile forward. However, retrograde and simultaneous contractions also occur to some extent in healthy individuals. The sphincter of Oddi is not an absolute barrier, so even during fasting there is a small quantity of bile that enters the duodenum.

Sphincter of Oddi dysmotility may impair entry of bile and/or pancreatic juice into the duodenum and lead to functional obstruction.

The neurohormonal regulation of the sphincter of Oddi activity is still poorly understood, but cholecystokinin is known to inhibit the sphincter of Oddi and thus enhance the flow of bile into the duodenum.

The integrated motor function of the gallbladder and the sphincter of Oddi plays an important role in regulating the enterohepatic circulation of bile

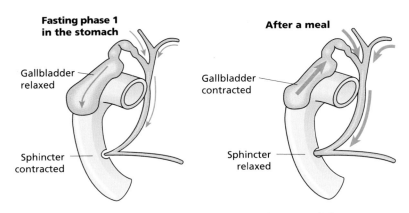

Figure 4.17 Bile flow in the biliary tree in the fasting and postprandial state.

acids. The sphincter of Oddi is also believed to play a role in the prevention of reflux from the duodenum.

Etiology
- Secondary to other diseases such as systemic sclerosis, diabetes mellitus, CIIP
- Drug-induced motility disorders e.g. opiates (see Table 4.2)
- Idiopathic.

Table 4.2 Drugs affecting sphincter of Oddi tone.

Increase sphincter tone
   opiates
   cholinergic agonists
   alpha-adrenergic agonists
   H_1-agonists

Decrease sphincter tone
   beta-agonists
   anticholinergic agents
   nitrates
   calcium antagonists

Symptoms
Epigastric pain and/or:
- abdominal (right upper quadrant) pain with or without radiation to the back
- dyspepsia-like symptom
- postcholecystectomy syndrome
- recurrent acute idiopathic pancreatitis.

Differential diagnosis
- Choledocholithiasis (ductal stones)—the most common cause of obstruction
- Papillitis—the inflammation and swelling of the papilla
- Papillary stenosis—can result from inflammation and subsequent scarring of the papilla of Vater with secondary damage of the sphincter of Oddi relaxatory mechanism
- Cancer—ampullary tumors, pancreatic carcinoma
- Chronic pancreatitis
- Irritable bowel syndrome.

Diagnostic procedures
Laboratory analysis
Laboratory tests (e.g. liver enzymes) should be taken to detect any laboratory signs of obstruction.

Ultrasonography

Commonly applied as the first-line investigation. It is highly reliable in the detection of stones in the gallbladder but the sensitivity is lower for the detection of stones in the common bile duct.

It is, however, possible to detect dilatation of the ductal system which could imply flow obstruction.

Dynamic ultrasonography can also be used for the detection of sphincter of Oddi dyskinesia. An increase in the common bile duct diameter of 1 mm or more in response to cholecystokinin or a fatty meal is suggestive of sphincter of Oddi dyskinesia.

Endoscopic retrograde cholangiopancreatography

Endoscopic retrograde cholangiopancreatography (ERCP) is the most sensitive method for evaluation of both pancreatic and biliary systems; and can reveal structural anomalies or abnormalities. Sphincter of Oddi dyskinesia is suggested by delayed drainage of contrast from the common bile duct (>45 min) and dilatation of the bile duct (>12 mm) during ERCP.

Biliary scintigraphy

The criterion for the possible diagnosis of dysfunction is a delay in the drainage of the intravenously administered radionuclide (Tc-HIDA) from the hepatic hilum into the duodenum.

Manometry

Sphincter of Oddi manometry is performed by endoscopically directing a motility catheter into the common bile or pancreatic duct with subsequent withdrawal into the high pressure zone of the sphincter (see Section 8.14).

Manometry remains the gold standard for the definition of sphincter of Oddi dysfunction (Fig. 4.18). Manometric findings suggestive of sphincter of Oddi dysmotility include:

- elevated basal sphincter of Oddi pressure—greater than 40 mmHg above the duodenal pressure
- an increased choledochoduodenal pressure gradient
- increased frequency of phasic contractions—greater than 10/min

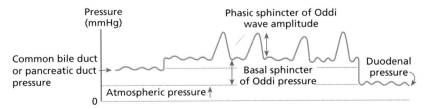

Figure 4.18 Sphincter of Oddi pressure profile demonstrating the features relevant to manometric recording.

- predominance of retrograde propagating waves (over 50% of the time)
- paradoxical increase in sphincter pressure in response to cholecystokinin
- increased amplitude of phasic contractions—greater than 200–300 mmHg.

Of these, an elevated basal pressure is the most discriminatory; the relative importance of these other criteria has not been defined.

A summary of the diagnostic work-up in patients with suspected sphincter of Oddi dysfunction is shown in Fig. 4.19.

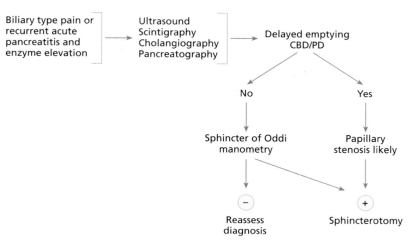

Figure 4.19 Diagnostic work-up in patient with suspected sphincter of Oddi dysfunction.

4.6 Sphincter of Oddi incompetence

Division of the sphincter of Oddi may lead to air and/or duodenal contents refluxing into the biliary tree, causing inflammation or infection of the ducts. Creation of a bacterial reservoir may in rare instances become symptomatic ("sump syndrome").

Manometric findings
- Disappearance of phasic contractions
- Disappearance of choledochoduodenal pressure gradient.

Transient sphincter of Oddi incompetence
This condition may occur if there are calculi migrating from the common bile duct into the duodenum.

5 Colonic and Anorectal Disorders

5.1 Physiology of the colon and anorectum

Functions of the colon

The functions of the colon are to:
- Absorb water and electrolytes that have entered the intestines with the digestive juices
- Transport waste products toward the rectum
- Temporarily store waste products in the sigmoid and descending colon.

The contractions and the flow of the colon are very slow, complex, and irregular in comparison to other gastrointestinal viscera. The flow of luminal contents through the colon is not uniformly progressive. There is antegrade and retrograde movement of the luminal contents.

It is disputed whether the periodic motor activity of the migrating motor complex (MMC), from the lower esophagus to the terminal ileum, propagates into the colon.

NONCYCLIC MOTOR EVENTS
The noncyclic features of colonic motility include irregular alternation of:
- Quiescence
- Nonpropagating contractions—these are segmental and stir the surface of the fecal mass in some way facilitating the absorption of fluid and electrolytes. These contractions may move contents over short distances in any direction. They last for seconds to minutes and are paced by the electrical slow waves of the colon
- Propagating contractions—these include high-amplitude propagated contractions (HAPC) which start in the ascending colon and move toward the sigmoid. These are thought to move the waste toward the rectum. The fecal mass rests in one place for a long period of time, but when these contractions occur, it moves forward abruptly and quickly for a short distance. (Definition of HAPC: amplitude over 80 mmHg, duration greater than 10 s, and propagation over at least 30 cm.)

The HAPC are associated with mass movements (Figs 5.1 & 5.2), a term used to describe the movement of stool, gas, or barium contrast over long colonic distances. HAPCs occur approximately twice a day in a normal unprepared colon and 4–6 times/day in a colon cleansed by cathartics.

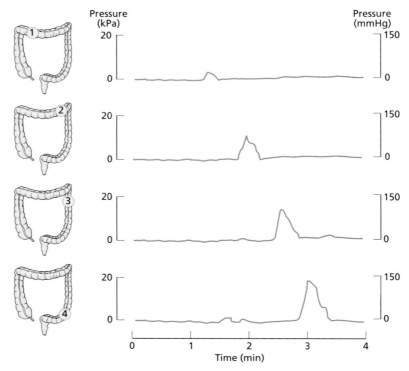

Figure 5.1 Mass movement in the colon.

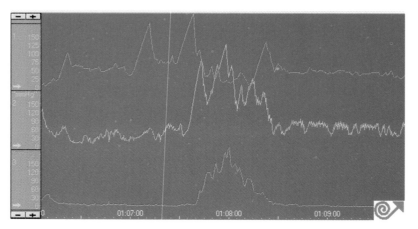

Figure 5.2 Propagating mass movement in the colon. The tracing shows a large pressure wave propagating through the transverse colon.

Other propagating contractions may propel fecal material over shorter distances.

CYCLIC MOTOR EVENTS (Fig. 5.3)

Cyclic colonic motility occurs only distal to the rectosigmoid junction.

The rectal motor complex (RMC) is a cyclic motor event in the rectum but is not synchronous with the MMC.

The RMC occurs every 90–300 min during the day and every 50–90 min at night and lasts an average of 10 min. Each complex comprises phasic contractions at a frequency of 3–4 min; the frequency of the electrical slow waves in this region.

Unlike the MMC the RMC is not abolished by feeding. This could be due to the colon being continuously in a digestive state and seldom empty.

The physiologic role of the RMC is still unknown, though it has been suggested that it may help to keep the rectum empty, especially at night.

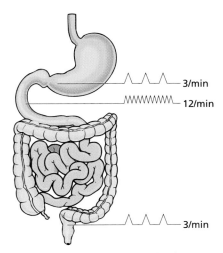

3/min

12/min

3/min

Figure 5.3 The rhythm of slow waves in the stomach, duodenum, and rectum.

GASTROCOLIC REFLEX

Eating stimulates colonic motility and results in an increase of colonic contractions which may provoke an urge to defecate. This is called the gastrocolonic response or gastrocolic reflex and occurs 20–40 min after beginning a meal. Despite its name, the gastrocolic reflex is not a true reflex since it is hormonally mediated. The colonic response is initiated by contact between the meal and the mucosa of the stomach and/or small intestine.

Function of the rectum

The main function of the rectum is to act as a reservoir of stool for short periods of time. This allows defecation to occur voluntarily at the appropriate time.

Functions of the anal canal

- Maintain fecal continence
- Control defecation.

Continence involves:

- detection of rectal contents
- discrimination of rectal contents
- voluntary and subconscious retention of rectal contents
- controlled expulsion of rectal contents.

Continence is maintained by the resting tone and reflex activity of the internal and external anal sphincters together with the muscles of the pelvic floor (Fig. 5.4).

The internal anal sphincter (IAS) is under autonomic control and is primarily responsible for resting tone.

The external anal sphincter (EAS) and the pelvic floor with the puborectalis sling are under voluntary control. These muscles also undergo a reflex contraction when intraabdominal pressure suddenly rises (for example, when sneezing or coughing).

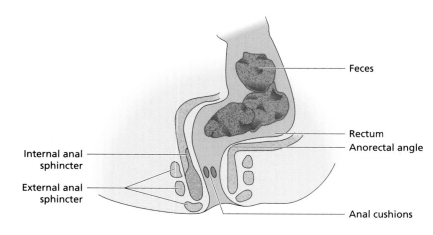

- Capacious and distensible rectum
- Firm, bulky feces
- Normal anorectal angle
- Normal anal canal and sphincter functions
- Anal cushions

Figure 5.4 Factors necessary for anal continence.

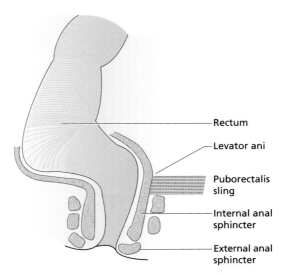

Rectum

Levator ani

Puborectalis
sling

Internal anal
sphincter

External anal
sphincter

Figure 5.5 Anatomy of the anorectum.

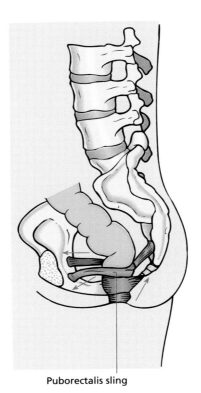

Puborectalis sling

Figure 5.6 The puborectalis sling.

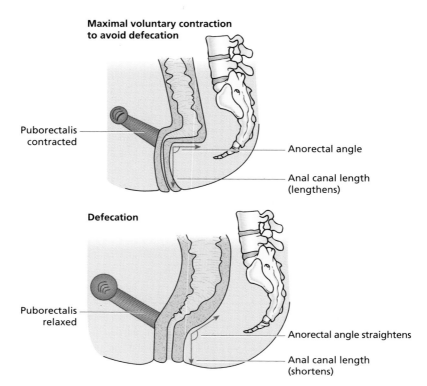

Figure 5.7 The anorectal angle.

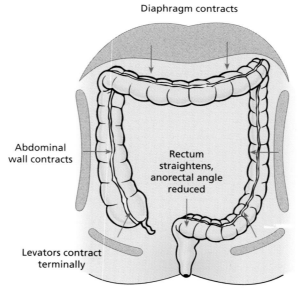

Figure 5.8 Mechanisms of defecation.

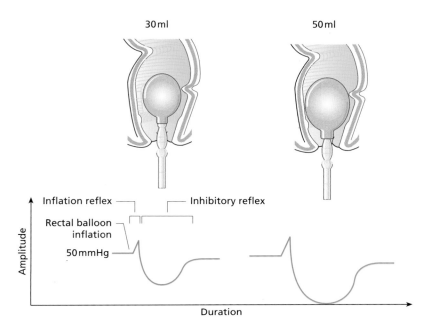

Figure 5.9 The rectoanal inhibitory reflex. Distention of the rectum leads to reflex relaxation of the EAS. The greater the distention, the greater the relaxation.

Contraction of the puborectalis sling is important in maintaining continence since it increases the anorectal angle, elevates the pelvic floor, and elongates the anal canal (Figs 5.5 & 5.6).

PHYSIOLOGY OF DEFECATION
For most people, defecation is often triggered by the gastrocolic reflex. Feces and gas in the colon are then transported to the rectum by peristaltic mass contractions, initiated by a meal.

Distention of the rectum is registered in the cerebral cortex and the reflex relaxation of the IAS occurs (the rectoanal inhibitory reflex (RAIR)) (see Fig. 5.9). As a consequence of the latter, the waste moves further down and comes into contact with receptors in the upper part of the anal canal. The receptors determine the quality of the content (the sampling reflex). If the time is right for defecation, impulses are sent to further contract the rectal muscles, relax the EAS and the pelvic floor with the puborectalis sling, to facilitate defecation.

Relaxation of the puborectalis sling produces a widening of the anorectal angle (normally 60–105°, increases to 140°) producing an unobstructed anal pathway which facilitates defecation (Figs 5.7 & 5.8).

If defecation has to be suppressed, a voluntary contraction of the EAS and pelvic floor, using the puborectalis sling, propels the luminal contents back up again above the rectum and the urge to defecate ceases.

5.2 Irritable bowel syndrome

Irritable bowel syndrome (IBS) is a common cause of abdominal pain. Fifty to seventy per cent of all patients who seek medical attention for gastro-intestinal problems are given a diagnosis of IBS.

The diagnosis of IBS is entirely clinical and is based on the combination of abdominal pain and altered bowel habit.

The diagnosis is usually made after all structural and biochemical causes of intestinal dysfunction have been excluded. However, the need for an extensive evaluation is often not necessary if a thorough patient history is taken.

Etiology

A variety of abnormalities of gastrointestinal function have been associated with symptoms of IBS:

* motility disturbances of the small bowel and the colon (Fig. 5.10)
* disturbed visceral perception.

In IBS the motor response to psychologic stress and food intake is often exaggerated and may precipitate symptoms.

Several other factors such as circulating hormones, diet and medications, and distention of intestinal segments, may also contribute to intestinal hyperreactivity in the intestines.

Distention of the bowel and rectum in patients with IBS tends to induce abdominal pain and discomfort at a much lower volume and pressure than in healthy individuals (Fig. 5.11).

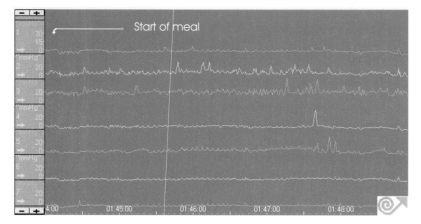

Figure 5.10 Colonic motility tracing in a patient with IBS. Pathological colon response with contractions of increasing frequency and increasing pressure postpran-dially have been seen in IBS patients compared to normal patients.

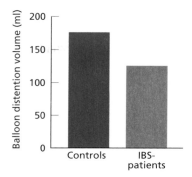

Figure 5.11 Pain perception in normal patients compared to patients with IBS. IBS-patients show a low tolerance to pain produced by balloon distention in the recto-sigmoid region compared to normals.

Symptoms
- Abdominal pain/discomfort that is often relieved by defecation or associated with a change in frequency/consistency of the stool
- Bloating or feeling of abdominal distention
- Disturbed defecation such as
  (a) altered stool frequency
  (b) altered stool form (lumpy/hard or loose/watery)
  (c) altered stool passage (straining or urgency, feeling of incomplete evacuation)
- Rectal fullness
- Nausea
- Early satiety.

Differential diagnosis
- Mechanical obstruction in the intestines (e.g. colorectal carcinoma)
- Ulcerative colitis, Crohn's disease
- Peptic ulcer disease
- Giardiasis
- Gluten-sensitive enteropathy
- Carbohydrate intolerance (e.g. lactose, sorbitol)
- Pseudoobstruction
- Gynecological disorders (e.g. endometriosis, pelvic inflammatory disease, ovarian carcinoma).

Diagnostic procedures
DIAGNOSTIC SYMPTOM CRITERIA
The diagnosis of IBS is made upon the combined symptoms according to the Rome criteria (a commonly employed schema):

99

- at least 3 months of continuous or recurrent symptoms of abdominal pain/discomfort that is often relieved by defecation and is associated with a change in frequency and/or consistency of the stool together with
- two or more of the following symptoms, occurring on at least 25% of the time or instances of defecation:

(a) altered stool frequency (for research purposes "altered" may be defined as more than three bowel movements each day or less than three bowel movements each week)

(b) altered stool form (lumpy/hard or loose/watery stool)

(c) altered stool passage (straining, urgency, or feeling of incomplete evacuation)

(d) passage of mucus

(e) bloating or feeling of abdominal distention.

VISCERAL STIMULATOR AND BAROSTAT

Visceral stimulators/barostats are computer controlled devices which make it possible to deliver precise, reproducible and automated stimuli for volume or pressure distention of the colon/rectum.

The test makes it possible to determine if there is an abnormal reaction to distention of the colon/rectum and to assess sensitivity thresholds in the colon and rectum (see Section 8.11).

Some of the abnormalities that may be found in IBS patients are:

- Increased sensitivity to colonic and rectal distention. Rectal distention in IBS patients seems to be associated with pain at lower volume and lower pressure level compared to asymptomatic healthy patients
- Increased tendency of spasm in the rectosigmoid region postprandially or after distention of intestinal segments.

5.3 Constipation

Etiology

Constipation is a common and distressing problem. It may be secondary to many diseases, or it may also be idiopathic.

Depending on the etiology, constipation may be divided into two main groups: colorectal and extracolonic constipation.

COLORECTAL CONSTIPATION

This consists of impaired colonic transport function.

- Secondary to structural abnormalities such as:

(a) volvulus

(b) strictures

(c) disorders of enteric nervous system (Hirschsprung's disease)

(d) tumors

- Outlet obstruction

- Colonic inertia—slow transit constipation. This is typically a lifelong and laxative-dependent form of constipation that mainly affects women. Colonic transit time is prolonged. There are no signs of rectal constipation.

EXTRACOLONIC CONSTIPATION
- Constipation secondary to systemic diseases such as:
  (a) hypothyroidism
  (b) diabetes mellitus
- Secondary to neurologic diseases such as:
  (a) multiple sclerosis
  (b) cerebral injury
  (c) spinal cord injury
  (d) peripheral denervation
  (e) Parkinson's disease
- Secondary to psychological factors such as:
  (a) depression
  (b) psychosis
  (c) anorexia nervosa
  (d) sexual abuse
- Secondary to medication such as:
  (a) anticholinergics
  (b) some antacids
  (c) antidepressants
  (d) iron
  (e) opiates
  (f) certain laxatives
- Secondary to patient immobilization
- Secondary to deficient diet
- Secondary to poor bowel habits.

Symptoms
- Problems emptying the bowel even though the urge to defecate is present
- Straining at defecation
- The consistency of the stool is lumpy and/or hard
- Infrequent defecation, less than three bowel movements in a week
- Sensation of incomplete evacuation.

Colorectal constipation due to outlet obstruction
In constipation due to outlet obstruction, the urge to defecate is preserved, but defecation is difficult and requires straining.

Outlet-type constipation may be due to morphologic defects or may be functional in origin.

Etiology

MORPHOLOGIC CAUSES OF OUTLET OBSTRUCTION

Rectal intussusception/rectal prolapse (Fig. 5.12)

An intussusception of the anterior rectal wall or a rectal prolapse may cause a mechanical obstruction of the opening of the anal canal making it impossible to defecate.

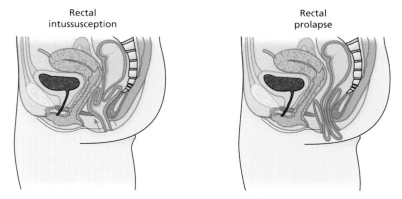

Figure 5.12 Rectal intussusception and rectal prolapse.

Rectocele (Fig. 5.13)

A rectocele may be of any size and is often asymptomatic. Rectoceles are common in women who have given birth. There is a defect in the recto-vaginal septa leading to protrusion into the vagina. Fecal mass can gather and lead to outlet obstruction.

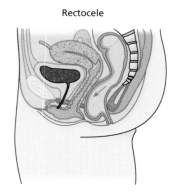

Figure 5.13 Rectocele.

FUNCTIONAL CAUSES OF OUTLET OBSTRUCTION

Spastic pelvic floor syndrome—anismus (Fig. 5.14)

This syndrome is characterized by a paradoxic contraction of the EAS and puborectalis muscle when the patient strains to defecate. This makes defecation impossible, since the anal canal is functionally closed off.

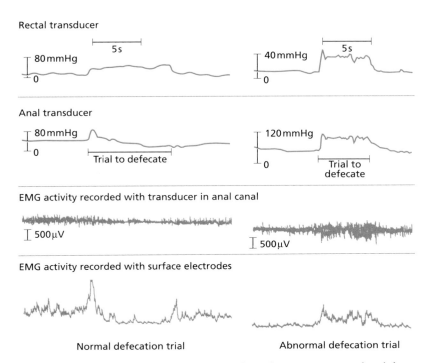

Rectal transducer

Anal transducer

EMG activity recorded with transducer in anal canal

EMG activity recorded with surface electrodes

Normal defecation trial   Abnormal defecation trial

Figure 5.14 Normal defecation versus pelvic floor dyssynergia. Reproduced from Schuster, 1993 with the permission of Williams & Wilkins.

Using electromyography (EMG), it is possible to record a paradoxic increase in activity in the puborectalis muscle and the EAS while straining to defecate.

Prolapse of the anterior wall while straining against a paradoxically contracted puborectalis muscle may result in the development of an ulcer as the anterior wall is compressed against the upper border of the internal anal sphincter. This is called the solitary rectal ulcer syndrome.

Hirschsprung's disease (see Section 6.6)
In Hirschsprung's disease the RAIR is absent due to congenital aganglionosis. Certain areas of the distal bowel do not receive enteric innervation causing a narrowed and spastic bowel, whereas the normally innervated proximal bowel is dilated and filled with fecal material. The IAS does not relax in order to defecate which causes outlet obstruction.

Descending perineum syndrome (Fig. 5.15)
The pudendal nerve which innervates the pelvic floor has been damaged, often due to vaginal delivery or straining against a tight anus over a long period of time. Pudendal neuropathy causes the pelvic floor to descend.

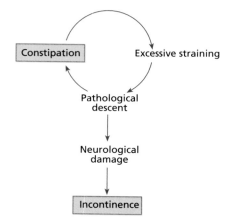

Figure 5.15 Descending perineum syndrome causing constipation and fecal incontinence.

This may cause outlet obstruction. In the long run, however, the descending perineum syndrome may lead to fecal incontinence since pudendal neuropathy also leads to impaired control of the EAS.

Symptoms in patients with constipation due to outlet obstruction

- Constant or frequent urge to defecate
- Straining
- Tenesmus
- Infrequent bowel movements
- Anorectal and perineal pain
- Feeling of incomplete evacuation
- Manual extraction of waste needed.

Differential diagnosis

- Proctitis
- Anorectal/colonic cancer
- Anal stenosis
- Ulcers from mechanical trauma (e.g. thermometers/enemas).

Diagnostic procedure (Fig. 5.16)

Digital rectal examination

Basic investigation with which structural abnormalities may be identified.

The perineal skin should also be stroked gently with a pin to elicit the anal wink reflex. This reflex is lost if the afferent or efferent nerves to or from the spinal cord have been damaged.

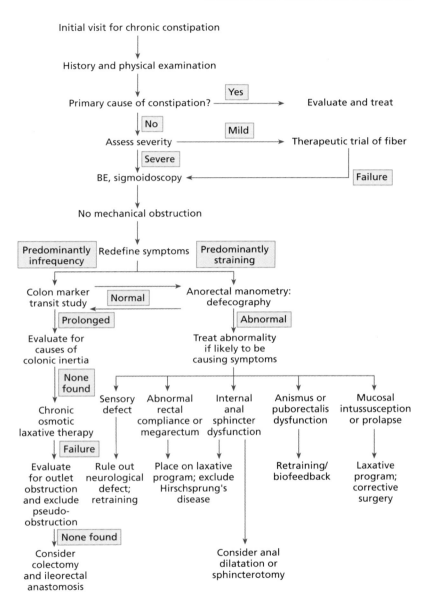

Figure 5.16 Algorithm for clinical approach to patients with chronic constipation. BE, barium enema. Reproduced from Champion M.C. & Orr W.C. (eds) *Evolving Concepts in Gastrointestinal Motility*. 1996, Blackwell Science, Oxford.

Clinical laboratory tests

These can detect primary processes which cause constipation (e.g. hypercalcemia, diabetes, hypothyroidism, hypokalemia).

Radiography

Plain radiograms of the abdomen will distinguish between fecal loading of the colon and gaseous distention. A barium enema can help to exclude mechanical obstruction, define megacolon, and analyze the pattern of haustral folds.

Proctosigmoidoscopy

This will provide direct visualization of the anal canal, rectum, and sigmoid, and identify obstruction, neoplasm, inflammation, infection, bleeding, hemorrhoidal prolapse, or fissures.

Colonoscopy

This will provide direct visualization of the entire colon and identify infectious disorders, inflammatory bowel diseases, and benign or malignant colorectal tumors.

Defecography

The rectum and the sigmoid are filled with barium paste. With fluoroscopy, it is possible to visualize the act of defecation and measure the anorectal angle and how it changes during defecation. It is also possible to measure the descent of the pelvic floor and visualize rectal prolapse, intussusception, rectocele, and functional outlet obstruction.

By using synchronized video manometry, the manometric recording can be simultaneously correlated with defecography.

Colonic transit time

The passage of radioopaque markers, ingested by the patient, can be followed on daily abdominal X-rays. In slow transit constipation, markers are typically retained throughout the colon whereas in outlet obstruction the markers will accumulate in the rectosigmoid region above the obstruction.

Expulsion test (balloon test)

This simple test estimates defecatory function. A water-filled balloon is inserted into the rectum. A normal individual should be able to expel a 150-ml balloon without difficulty.

Electromyography

By recording the electrical activity of the external sphincter and the puborectalis muscle, EMG can detect any paradoxic increase in activity in these muscle groups during defecation. This finding would support the diagnosis of anismus.

Pudendal nerve terminal motor latency

The function of the pudendal nerve (which innervates the pelvic floor and the EAS) can be determined by recording activity in the sphincters in response to transrectal stimulation of the motor nerve electrically. The time taken from the onset of stimulation to the first measurable contraction of the EAS is measured—this is the pudendal nerve terminal motor latency. If prolonged it indicates a pudendal neuropathy. Pudendal nerve damage has been frequently observed in patients with the descending perineum syndrome and also in patients with idiopathic fecal incontinence (see Section 8.13).

Anorectal manometry

This test provides information on anorectal muscle tone and the coordination between the rectum and the anal sphincters (see Section 8.10).

5.4 Fecal incontinence (Fig. 5.17)

Fecal incontinence is a symptom which may be secondary to many different causes.

The autonomically controlled IAS together with the voluntarily controlled EAS and pelvic floor muscles help to maintain fecal continence. If these structures or their neural input are damaged, there is a risk of fecal incontinence.

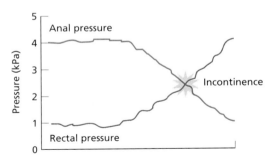

Figure 5.17 Fecal incontinence occurs when rectal pressure exceeds anal pressure.

Etiology

- Gastrointestinal: fecal impaction with overflow, ulcerative proctitis, rectal cancer, radiation proctitis, inflammatory bowel disease
- Neurologic: dementia, multiple sclerosis, spinal cord disease, stroke
- Metabolic: diabetes mellitus
- Traumatic: childbirth, anorectal surgery, sphincter trauma, sexual abuse

- Congenital abnormalities
- Idiopathic fecal incontinence.

Some patients with fecal incontinence have lost the sampling function of the anal canal. The patient cannot sense and "sample" what has passed into the anal canal and cannot therefore react to prevent incontinence. The anal sensitivity threshold provides an index of pudendal neuropathy.

A considerable proportion of patients with idiopathic fecal incontinence have been found to have damage to the motor portion of the pudendal nerve (pudendal neuropathy). This leads to impaired function of the EAS and the pelvic floor muscles which are of great importance in maintaining fecal continence. In those patients EAS contraction following rectal distention is often absent or occurs only at much higher distending volumes.

In inflammatory bowel disease rectal compliance is reduced and there is an intolerance to distention of the rectum at volumes that would not be sensed by normal individuals. They may, therefore, experience fecal incontinence, associated with urgency, despite normal anal sphincter function.

Rectal compliance may be impaired also in patients with idiopathic fecal incontinence. Compliance is important if the rectum is to serve as a fecal reservoir. The rectum must be distensible to accommodate incoming feces and thereby prevent incontinence.

Symptoms
MINOR INCONTINENCE
- Minor involuntary soiling
- Incontinence with flatus, or loose or watery stool.

MAJOR INCONTINENCE
- Poor control of solid formed stool
- Frequent and spontaneous evacuation of formed bowel movements.

Diagnostic procedures
MORPHOLOGIC DIAGNOSTICS
Digital rectal examination
This will identify structural abnormalities and also provide some assessment of basal sphincter tone and the squeeze response.

Proctosigmoidoscopy
This will provide direct visualization of the anal canal, rectum, and sigmoid and identify obstruction, neoplasm, inflammation, infection, bleeding, hemorrhoidal prolapse, or fissures.

Radiography
Barium enema will help to identify anatomic anomalies, infectious disorders, inflammatory bowel diseases and benign or malignant colorectal tumors.

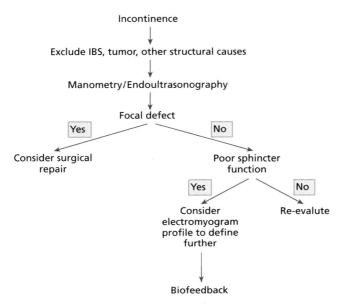

Figure 5.18 Algorithm for decision making in patients with fecal incontinence.

Colonoscopy

Can be used instead of radiography to identify anatomic anomalies, infectious disorders, inflammatory bowel diseases, and benign or malignant colorectal tumors.

Anorectal endosonography

Provides a detailed morphologic assessment of the IAS and EAS and can readily identify focal anatomic defects.

FUNCTIONAL DIAGNOSTICS (Fig. 5.18)

Anorectal manometry with vector volume analysis

Can be used to quantify the resistance to spontaneous defecation provided by the anorectal sphincter mechanism. The resting and squeeze pressures of the anal canal and the rectal inhibitory reflex are evaluated (see Section 8.10).

Some of the indications for using anorectal manometry in patients with fecal incontinence are:

- to evaluate the relative contributions of IAS and/or EAS dysfunction to fecal incontinence
- to document the baseline level of sphincter function prior to biofeedback training
- pre-/postoperative evaluation of anorectal sphincter repair.

Vector volume analysis provides an assessment of the radial distribution of pressure within the anal canal. It can identify a focal defect which can be helpful in guiding anorectal sphincter repair and also help in assessing the outcome.

Electromyography

EMG records the electrical activity of the EAS and puborectalis muscles. Contraction of these muscles is necessary to prevent incontinence. In biofeedback training one may use EMG recordings to visualize the activity of these muscles (see Section 8.12).

Pudendal nerve terminal motor latency

The function of the pudendal nerve (which innervates the pelvic floor and the EAS) can be determined by recording activity in the sphincters in response to transrectal stimulation of the motor nerve electrically. The time taken from the onset of stimulation to the first measurable contraction of the EAS is measured—this is the pudendal nerve terminal motor latency. If prolonged it indicates a pudendal neuropathy.

Pudendal neuropathy has been commonly identified in patients with idiopathic fecal incontinence (see Section 8.13).

5.5 Anal fissures

An anal fissure is a linear defect in the mucosa of the lower half of the anal canal extending from the anal verge toward the dentate line (Fig. 5.19).

A fissure often begins following an episode of either diarrhea or constipation. Some heal spontaneously; others, however, become chronic. As the distal end of the fissure lies in a region that has somatic innervation, pain may become intense following defecation.

Reflex spasm of the EAS occurs whenever the fissure is disturbed.

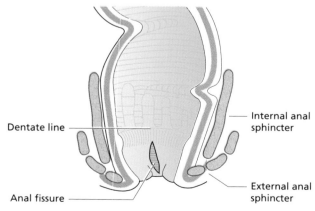

Dentate line

Internal anal sphincter

Anal fissure

External anal sphincter

Figure 5.19 Anal fissures—a vertical split in the squamous lined lower half of the anal canal.

Symptoms
- Wetting, leakage of anal secretions
- Hematochezia
- Pruritus, burning
- Mild to severe pain, which may or may not be associated with defecation
- Constipation due to pain associated with defecation.

Diagnostic procedures
MORPHOLOGIC DIAGNOSTICS
Digital rectal examination
Though capable of providing important information digital rectal examination is often impossible in a patient with a fissure because of pain.

Proctosigmoidoscopy
This will identify the location and extent of the fissure as well as any associated pathology.

FUNCTIONAL DIAGNOSTICS
Anorectal manometry
Manometry is not required for the diagnosis of anal fissure and is not routinely indicated.

If manometry is performed, some manometric abnormalities are present, such as:
- high resting anal sphincter pressures
- normal IAS relaxation and EAS contraction—IAS relaxation is often followed by an immediate "overshoot" contraction.

When fissures have been successfully treated, the "overshoot" contraction disappears.

6 Pediatric Gastrointestinal Problems

6.1 Gastroesophageal reflux

Regurgitation of gastric contents is very common in infants. This implies that the mechanisms that prevent gastroesophageal reflux are not completely developed at birth but mature during infancy. A gradual maturation of the lower esophageal sphincter (LES) pressure has been documented in the first 3 months of life. The abdominal portion of the esophagus and the total length of the LES are shorter in newborns, but gradually lengthen during early infancy.

These anatomic and functional factors predispose to the regurgitation of stomach contents in young infants.

There is, however, a group of infants and children that suffers clinical consequences as a result of gastroesophageal reflux. The functional or physiologic reflux has to be separated therefore from clinical gastroesophageal reflux disease (GERD).

FUNCTIONAL GASTROESOPHAGEAL REFLUX

- Common in children under 6 months of age
- Effortless regurgitation
- Painless regurgitation mainly following eating
- Growth and development are not affected
- Regurgitation ceases as the child grows older.

GASTROESOPHAGEAL REFLUX DISEASE

GERD should be considered when the reflux leads to:

- persistent severe emesis
- failure to thrive
- recurrent pneumonia, apnea, asthma
- esophageal mucosa changes related to excessive exposure to gastric contents
- dystonia
- anemia.

Etiology

The etiology to pathological gastroesophageal reflux in children is basically the same as in adults (see Section 3.1). Most reflux episodes in children seem to occur during transient LES relaxations (TLESRs). The relaxations increase after feeding which suggests that distention of the stomach is a significant source of reflux in children (see Fig. 3.5). LES incompetence, impaired esophageal clearance and delayed gastric emptying are also important etiologic factors.

Symptoms

- Regurgitation, nausea, vomiting
- Failure to thrive
- Symptoms suggestive of anemia
- Recurrent aspiration causing pneumonia, apnea, or reactive airways disease
- Dystonia (Sandifer's syndrome).

Diagnostic procedures

The diagnostic procedures used in children to identify gastroesophageal reflux are mainly the same as in adults (Fig. 6.1). One must, however, bear in mind to only perform studies of great value for the diagnosis and treatment. (For 24-h pH monitoring in children, see Section 9.1.)

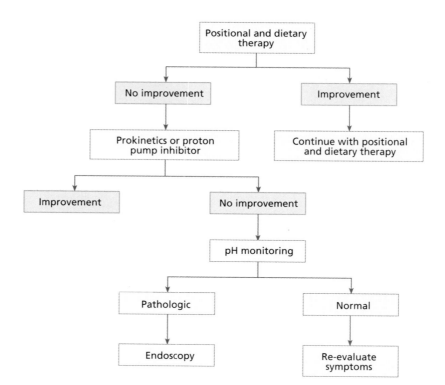

Figure 6.1 The clinical approach to the assessment of gastroesophageal reflux in children.

6.2 Respiratory problems

Gastroesophageal reflux may extend to reach the larynx and the bronchial tree which can cause respiratory problems (coughing, wheezing, stridor). Some therapeutic strategies for these symptoms (e.g. medications, such as theophylline, beta-adrenergic bronchodilators, or chest physiotherapy) may in themselves provoke reflux leading to even more exaggerated symptoms.

Symptoms

GERD-related respiratory problems in children may include:
- apneic episodes
- pulmonary aspiration which may cause pneumonia
- respiratory distress with signs of bronchospasm.

Differential diagnosis

- Apneic episodes:
  (a) sepsis, viral infection
  (b) neurologic abnormality, metabolic derangement (hypoglycaemia, hypocalcaemia)
  (c) idiopathic apnea of prematurity
  (d) reflex to laryngeal stimulation by milk
  (e) anatomic abnormality
  (f) uncoordinated feeding/breathing sequency
  (g) functional airways obstruction (tracheomalacia)
- Pulmonary aspiration:
  (a) swallowing incoordination
  (b) laryngeal cleft
  (c) tracheoesophageal fistula
- Bronchospasm:
  (a) viral infection
  (b) intrathoracic airways obstruction (foreign body)
  (c) primary lung disease
  (d) inhalation of irritants (cigarette smoke, dust)
  (e) congestive heart failure.

Diagnostic procedures

Diagnostic procedures to diagnose reflux causing respiratory symptoms in children, include:

Radionuclide gastroesophageal scintigram (milk scan)

Which utilizes radiolabeled milk to demonstrate if refluxed material is entering the lungs. This method, however, involves radiation exposure.

24-h pH-metry

Which allows long term pH measurements in the esophagus to detect acid reflux. In children this test may be especially valuable in linking symptoms to reflux episodes especially when combined with other respiratory polygraphic measurements including O_2 saturation, P_{CO_2}, P_{O_2}, and heart rate (see Section 9.1).

6

chapter

6.3 Esophageal motility disorders

Other than GER, disorders of esophageal motility in children are rare and include:

1 achalasia
2 collagen–vascular disease
3 neuromuscular disease.

1 Achalasia

Although this condition is uncommon at any age, fewer than 5% of those affected develop symptoms before the age of 15 years. In achalasia patients the LES becomes hypertensive and does not relax sufficiently to let food pass easily down into the stomach. There is also aperistalsis of the distal esophageal body in these patients.

Symptoms

- Progressive dysphagia (the most common symptom)
- Recurrent emesis
- Failure to thrive
- Respiratory symptoms.

Differential diagnosis

- Strictures
- Benign neoplasms
- Vascular rings
- Webs
- Foreign bodies
- Severe esophagitis (peptic, infectious, chemical, drug induced).

Diagnostic procedures

The diagnostic procedures used in children to identify achalasia are the same as in adults (e.g. radiography, manometry) see Section 9.2.

2 Collagen–vascular diseases

The esophagus can be affected in childhood by a number of collagen diseases such as:

(a) progressive systemic sclerosis (scleroderma)
(b) polymyositis/dermatomyositis
(c) mixed connective tissue disease.

Most children (75%) with scleroderma and mixed connective tissue diseases demonstrate esophageal motor abnormalities. These diseases, however, are rare in childhood.

(a) Scleroderma

The etiology of scleroderma is unknown, but it causes atrophy and sclerosis of esophageal smooth muscles, which leads to impaired peristalsis in the distal esophagus and LES incompetence.

Esophageal symptoms

Due to LES incompetence there is often severe GER leading to:
- heartburn
- regurgitation
- dysphagia
- chest pain.

Symptoms may, however, be relatively mild despite severe mucosal disease.

Diagnostic procedures

In order to detect sclerodermic involvement of the esophagus, manometry may be performed (see Section 9.2).

Manometric findings
- Low or absent LES pressure
- Weak or absent distal esophageal contractions and peristalsis
- Normal upper esophageal peristalsis and upper esophageal sphincter (UES).

(b) Polymyositis/dermatomyositis

Polymyositis is a chronic inflammatory myopathy of uncertain cause. When a skin rash is also present, it is termed dermatomyositis.

Since this disease affects striated muscle fibers, it causes muscular weakness and variable degrees of pain, swelling, or atrophy of affected muscles.

Vasculitis involving the skin and the gastrointestinal tract is also common in children with dermatomyositis.

Esophageal symptoms

The pharynx and the upper third of the esophagus, which consists of striated muscle fibers, will be affected leading to symptoms such as:
- aspiration
- nasopharyngeal regurgitation
- oropharyngeal dysphagia
- failure to thrive.

Diagnostic procedure

With esophageal manometry one may detect esophageal involvement of the disease (see Section 9.2).

Manometric findings (see Fig. 9.7)
- Normal LES pressure and relaxation
- Normal peristalsis in the distal esophageal body
- Decreased amplitude of peristalsis in the proximal esophagus
- An increase in the number of swallows which result in the development of simultaneous waves in the proximal esophagus.

(c) Mixed connective tissue diseases

This term describes a disorder in a group of patients who exhibit features of systemic lupus erythematosus (SLE), scleroderma, and polymyositis. These patients may exhibit any combination of several symptoms such as arthritis, fever, myositis, anemia, leukopenia, Raynaud's phenomenon, and esophageal motility abnormalities.

Esophageal symptoms

These are heartburn and regurgitation due to reflux.

Diagnostic procedures

With esophageal manometry one may detect esophageal involvement. The manometric findings are similar to those in scleroderma (see Section 9.2).

Manometric findings
- Decrease in LES pressure
- Decrease in distal esophageal peristalsis.

3 Neuromuscular diseases

Symptoms related to gastroesophageal reflux occur frequently in children with diseases of the central nervous system.

Some of these symptoms may be:
- recurrent vomiting
- pulmonary aspiration
- failure to thrive.

Symptoms may often be relatively silent despite advanced mucosal and extraesophageal disease.

SEVERE PSYCHOMOTOR RETARDATION
Manometric findings
UES and esophageal body abnormalities such as:
- decreased amplitude of peristalsis in the esophageal body
- abnormal motor response to swallows.

MUSCULAR DYSTROPHY

Muscular dystrophy includes a group of genetically determined myopathies characterized by progressive atrophy or degeneration of muscle cells. As these disorders involve skeletal muscles, pharyngeal and UES dysfunction and impaired motility in the proximal esophagus are common. In adults, involvement of esophageal smooth muscle may be prominent causing other symptoms (esophageal dysphagia and GERD).

Manometric findings
- Low amplitude peristaltic waves in the proximal esophagus
- Low UES pressure and pharyngeal peristalsis.

6.4 Pseudoobstruction

Chronic intestinal pseudoobstruction (CIP) refers to the child having symptoms of bowel obstruction but no mechanical obstructing lesion is present. In childhood primary forms of CIP, which are largely congenital, occur more commonly than secondary forms (for CIP classification see Section 4.4).

The majority of congenital forms of both neuropathic and myopathic pseudoobstruction are sporadic, i.e. there is no family history of CIP, no associated syndrome, and no predisposing factors such as toxins, infections, ischemia, or autoimmune disease.

Symptoms

The onset may be precipitous or slowly progressive. Symptoms at presentation may include:

- abdominal distention
- constipation
- vomiting
- failure to gain weight
- diarrhea due to bacterial overgrowth
- urologic abnormalities such as dilated, atonic bladder and ureters
- seizures
- temperature instability
- dysphagia
- burping
- flatus.

Some of the abnormalities that may be found by conventional radiologic studies and pH monitoring are:

- gastroesophageal reflux
- generalized dilatation of the small bowel
- delayed gastric emptying
- megaduodenum

Diagnostic procedures

To detect CIP the same diagnostic tools are used as in adults. This includes radiography to exclude mechanical obstructions, antroduodenal manometry (the most sensitive test for CIP), electrogastrography (EGG), and histopathologic evaluation of tissue samples (see Sections 4.4 & 9.3).

6

chapter

6.5 Constipation

Constipation is a symptom that can be associated with many different disorders.

Etiology

COLORECTAL CONSTIPATION DUE TO STRUCTURAL DISEASES OF THE ANUS, RECTUM, COLON, OR SMALL INTESTINE

- Aganglionosis (Hirschsprung's disease, see below; pseudoobstruction)
- Anal stenosis
- Anorectal malformation
- Idiopathic megarectum and megacolon (see below)
- Painful disorders of the anus (fissures, dermatitis)
- Outlet obstruction (e.g. anismus).

EXTRACOLONIC CONSTIPATION

Secondary to other diseases

- Endocrinologic, metabolic, and toxic (diabetes mellitus, hypothyroidism, etc.)
- Neurologic (spinal cord injury, myelomeningocele)
- Connective tissue disease (scleroderma, cystic fibrosis, SLE).

Secondary to psychiatric disorders

- Depression
- Anorexia nervosa
- Psychosis
- Sexual abuse.

Secondary to drugs and toxins

BEHAVIORAL DISORDERS

Child may hold back defecation, creating constipation.

Symptoms

- Reduced stool frequency
- Difficulty or delay in the passage of feces
- Firm, hard consistency of stool
- Fecal overflow soiling
- Abdominal pain
- Anorexia
- Vomiting
- Failure to thrive
- Abdominal distention
- Flatus.

Diagnostic procedures

In children with constipation, the same procedures as in adults are performed, e.g. abdominal radiography to define fecal loading, and anorectal manometry mainly to exclude Hirschsprung's disease (see Sections 5.3 & 9.5).

Some authorities also suggest that colonic manometry is especially useful in the assessment of constipation in children. The absence of high-amplitude propagated contractions (HAPCs) is predictive of severe colonic motor dysfunction (see Section 9.4).

6.6 Hirschsprung's disease

Etiology

Hirschsprung's disease, or congenital aganglionosis, is a congenital anomaly characterized by the absence of ganglion cells in the myenteric and sub-mucosal plexuses (see Fig. 1.3) of the affected segment. The bowel may be involved to a variable extent: from a short segment of the distal rectum to the entire colon and small intestine.

The aganglionic segment remains in a state of tonic uninhibited contraction and fails to relax, creating a functional obstruction. This often leads to dilatation of the proximal colon or intestine above the aganglionic segment.

Most commonly, Hirschsprung's disease affects the rectosigmoid region and symptoms begin at birth. Ninety five percent of infants with Hirschsprung's disease fail to pass meconium during the first 24 h of birth. Most children are diagnosed within their first year, but some cases are not recognized until the ages of 3–12 years.

Ultrashort segment Hirschsprung's disease is an uncommon condition that involves only the very distal rectum. This condition is usually diagnosed much later and its recognition can even be delayed into adult life.

Symptoms
- Constipation
- Symptoms of intestinal obstruction
- Vomiting
- Abdominal distention
- Weight loss
- Failure to thrive.

Diagnostic procedures
Radiography
Colonic X-ray with a carefully performed barium enema can reveal the transition zone between the distal aganglionic narrowed segment with its characteristic "saw tooth" contractions and the proximal dilated segment. However, this test is not accurate enough since there is a high incidence of false-positive and false-negative tests.

6

chapter

Biopsy

Suction rectal biopsies represent the gold standard for the diagnosis of Hirschsprung's disease in infants and young children. Biopsies from the contracted segment of the bowel, stained for acetylcholinesterase, will reveal an absence of ganglion cells and hyperplastic neural elements in the myenteric and the submucosal plexus.

In ultrashort segment Hirschsprung's disease, biopsies may miss the aganglionic zone, and anorectal manometry becomes the only way to establish the diagnosis.

Anorectal manometry (Fig. 6.2)

In children with Hirschsprung's disease, the response of the internal anal sphincter to rectal balloon distention is abnormal. The rectoanal inhibitory

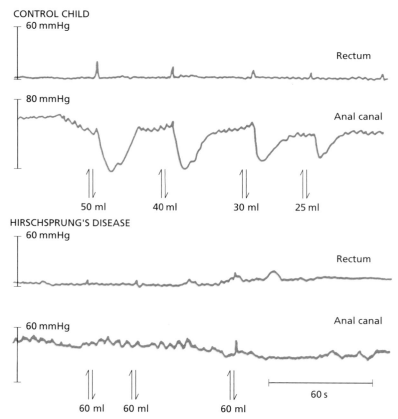

Figure 6.2 Tracings from a patient with Hirschsprung's disease. The double arrows indicate distention of a rectal balloon with air for 1 s which results in decreased anal pressure (the RAIR) in the control child but not in the child with Hirschsprung's disease. Reproduced from Hyman, 1994. Courtesy of Academic Professional Information Services Inc., New York, NY.

reflex is absent resulting in the absence of internal anal sphincter relaxation on distention of the rectum (see Section 9.5).

6.7 Megacolon/megarectum

Megacolon/megarectum is a descriptive term for dilatation of the colon/rectum (Fig. 6.3).

In constipation the retention of solid fecal material in the rectum and/or colon may distend the rectum and result in megarectum. Dilatation of the rectum in itself leads to large amounts of stool being required to stretch the walls of the rectum to assess the urge of defecation. In a high capacity rectum, the rectoanal inhibitory reflex becomes insensitive. Larger balloon inflation volumes will be required to detect the reflex.

When the stool is stored for a long time in the rectum, it becomes hard and painful to defecate. The child tries to avoid defecation, perpetuating a vicious cycle with even more stool gathering in the colon/rectum.

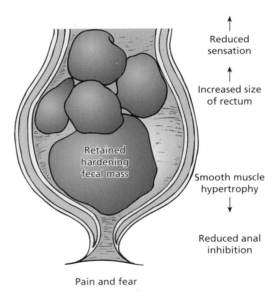

↑
Reduced
sensation

↑
Increased size
of rectum

Retained
hardening
fecal mass

Smooth muscle
hypertrophy

↓

Reduced anal
inhibition

Pain and fear

Figure 6.3 Pathophysiology of megarectum. Reproduced from Milla, 1988 with permission. Copyright John Wiley & Sons Limited.

Classification of megacolon/megarectum
CONGENITAL OR NEUROGENIC
Colonic dilatation results from functional obstruction of the rectum which is the case in Hirschsprung's disease.

ACQUIRED OR PSYCHOGENIC
This can be secondary to any of the many causes of constipation.

Symptoms
- See symptoms of constipation, p. 120
- Fecal soiling is very common.

DIAGNOSTIC PROCEDURES
Abdominal radiography
Demonstrates the degree of fecal loading and distention of the rectum/colon.

6.8 Fecal incontinence

The age at which fecal soiling begins to be considered inappropriate varies among different cultures. Fecal incontinence in a child should, however, not be considered a medical problem before the age of three. The age when treatment is initiated may be later depending on the cultural context.

Functional incontinence occurs more frequently in boys (four times as much) than in girls. The difference is thought to be due to the fact that boys often urinate while standing and do not, therefore, take additional time necessary to defecate in the toilet. When girls squat to urinate they are more likely to pass stools at the same time.

Encopresis is a term used to distinguish children with functional incontinence from those with incontinence resulting from neurologic injury or malformations of the anal canal.

Etiology
FECAL IMPACTION (Fig. 6.4)
This is the most common cause of incontinence in children. Various studies have shown that as many as 97% of instances of functional incontinence in

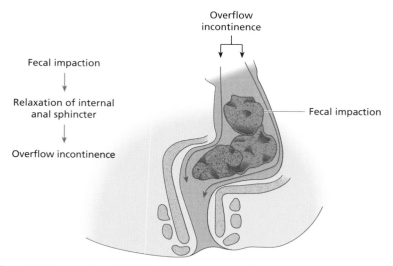

Overflow
incontinence

Fecal impaction
↓
Relaxation of internal
anal sphincter
↓
Overflow incontinence

Fecal impaction

Figure 6.4 Impacted stools in the rectum causing overflow incontinence.

children are due to fecal impaction. This constipation was in turn often associated with pelvic floor dyssynergia (anismus).

DECREASED ANORECTAL SENSITIVITY

This may contribute to incontinence by causing the reflex inhibition of the internal anal sphincter to occur before the patient perceives the presence of stool in the rectum. It may also exacerbate constipation by decreasing the frequency and intensity of the urge to defecate. The changes in sensory threshold may be a consequence of fecal impaction which may alter the tone and viscoelastic properties of the bowel wall.

NEUROLOGIC CAUSES

These include spinal cord disease, especially low spinal cord and cauda equina lesions, and brain lesions.

CONGENITAL ABNORMALITIES

These include malformation of the anal canal.

TRAUMATIC CAUSES

These include sphincter trauma and anorectal surgery.

BEHAVIORAL DISORDER

Fear of the toilet, or an effort to acquire control over or attention of parents. Recently, theories based on psychological etiology have been disputed. Instead, the psychological symptoms seen in incontinent children are thought to be a consequence of their soiling.

METABOLIC DISORDERS

Diabetes mellitus may lead to a decrease in rectal sensitivity and spontaneous transient internal anal sphincter relaxations.

Symptoms

Involuntary fecal soiling.

Diagnostic procedures

The same diagnostic procedures are performed in children with fecal incontinence as in adults (see Section 5.4).

In order to perform pH-metry, motility recordings, and a variety of other diagnostic sampling and testing in the gastrointestinal tract, it is necessary to intubate catheters nasally or orally.

The optimal catheter should be small enough in diameter, flexible, wetable, and biocompatible so that intubation is easily performed and that the catheter is comfortable for the patient during the study.

7.1 Catheters

Catheters for pH-metry (Fig. 7.1)

ANTIMONY CATHETERS

Advantages of disposable antimony catheters
- Internal reference
- Small diameters
- No risk for cross-contamination
- Easy to intubate.

Advantages of multiuse antimony catheters
- Small diameters
- Cost effective
- Easy to intubate.

Disadvantages of antimony catheters
- Not recommended for gastric studies
- Less reliable than glass and ion-sensitive field effect transistor (ISFET) catheters
- They require phosphate-free buffer for calibration.

ISFET CATHETERS

Advantages
- Not fragile
- Rapid response
- Recommended for esophageal and gastric studies
- Dry storage
- Cost effective
- Easy to introduce
- Capable of recording from multiple sites with a single catheter
- Can be combined with pressure sensors in the same catheter.

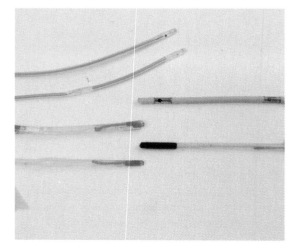

Figure 7.1 Different types of catheters for pH monitoring. *From top to bottom*: Zinetics 24M multiuse antimony pH catheter; Synectics multiuse antimony pH catheter; ISFET pH catheter; disposable antimony catheter with internal reference and infusion port from Zinetics; glass pH catheter from Ingold; disposable antimony catheter with internal reference from Zinetics.

Disadvantages
- New technique
- Somewhat higher initial cost
- External reference.

GLASS CATHETERS
Advantages
- Internal reference
- Recommended for esophageal and gastric studies.

Disadvantages
- Fragile
- Expensive
- Wet storage
- Cross-contamination risk
- The tip of the catheter is very stiff which makes it more difficult to intubate
- Only one sensor per catheter.

Catheters for motility recordings (Fig. 7.2)

These catheters are of two basic types: the water-perfused and the solid state catheters. The water-perfused catheters have multiple lumens within the catheter. Each opening (port) on the catheter has its own lumen to record pressure changes at this point. The number of ports and the configuration of the catheters varies and depend on what study they should be used for. The water-perfused catheter requires a pneumohydraulic infusion pump to generate a constant pressure and flow rate through each lumen of the catheter. Each individual lumen of the catheter has to be connected to the external pressure transducer where the pressure increase is converted to an electrical signal.

The solid state catheters have miniature strain gauge transducers built into the catheter, so that pressure changes directly influence the transducers to generate electrical output signals.

WATER-PERFUSED MULTILUMEN CATHETERS
Advantages
- Cost effective
- Allows the user considerable flexibility in configuring individual catheters in terms of number of and interval between recording ports.

Disadvantages
- Mainly for stationary studies
- Slow response rate
- Less suitable for upper esophageal sphincter (UES) studies.

SOLID STATE CATHETERS
Advantages
- Fast response
- Can be used in an ambulatory setting
- No water perfusion required
- Easy to use and to calibrate.

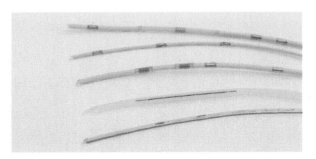

Figure 7.2 Different types of esophageal manometry catheters. *From top to bottom*: the "Golden standard" solid state sphinctometer catheter; the three-channel solid state catheter; the "Castell type" solid state catheter; the water-perfused Dentsleeve catheter for esophageal manometry; the water-perfused pediatric motility catheter (PMC) from Zinetics.

Disadvantages
- Expensive
- Limited number of sensors (too many will increase the outer diameter of the catheter)
- Fragile
- Functional lifespan dependent on how the catheter is treated, both in use and in cleaning.

SLEEVE CATHETER AND SPHINCTOMETER (Fig. 7.2)

Both catheters are intended for measuring sphincter resting tone and relaxation. The sleeve catheter is water-perfused and has, for LES measurements, a 6 cm longitudinal membrane which records the maximum pressure obtained at any part of the sensor.

The newly developed sphinctometer has a 6 cm long circumferential solid state sensor which records the average sphincter pressure.

Advantage
Since the sleeve and sphinctometer cover a long distance there is little risk for dislocation of the sensor in the LES or UES.

Other specific probes (Fig. 7.3)

BILIRUBIN-SENSITIVE PROBE

The fiberoptic probe emits light at a wavelength of 453 nm. Bile reflux contains bilirubin which has a characteristic absorption peak at the same wavelength. The probe may be used to detect bilirubin as the emitted light signal of the specific wavelength is absorbed proportionally to the bilirubin concentration.

CADMIUM–TELLURIDE PROBE FOR GASTRIC-EMPTYING STUDIES

This is an isotope-sensitive probe which is nasally placed in the stomach or the duodenum to record the passage of a radiolabeled meal.

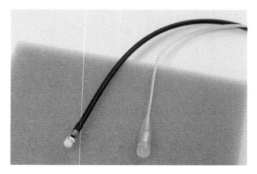

Figure 7.3 The fiberoptic probe for bile reflux studies (*left*) and the gamma probe for ambulatory gastric emptying studies (*right*).

7.2 Nasal intubation

Contraindications

- Nasopharyngeal or upper esophageal obstruction
- Severe uncontrolled coagulopathy
- Severe maxillofacial trauma and/or basilar skull fracture
- Bullous disorders of the esophageal mucosa
- Patient with cardiac instability or other conditions in whom vagal stimulation is poorly tolerated.

Relative contraindications

- Recent gastric surgery
- Esophageal tumors or ulcers
- Esophageal varices
- Poor patient cooperation.

Complications

INTUBATION

- Nasal or pharyngeal trauma/hemorrhage
- Laryngeal trauma
- Nasotracheal intubation
- Esophageal or gastric trauma/perforation
- Vomiting
- Vasovagal syndrome
- Bronchospasm
- Trigger trigeminal neuralgia
- Introduction/transmission of infection.

EXTUBATION

- Mucosal damage
- Entrapment of catheter in viscus.

Equipment

- The catheter or probe required for the specific diagnostic procedure
- Water-soluble lubricant
- Anesthetic spray/jelly (e.g. Lidocaine)
- Glass of water with a straw
- Emesis basin and tissues and/or towel
- Disposable gloves.

Before the study

- No food or drink should be taken for at least 6 h prior to the intubation in order to avoid aspiration

chapter 7

131

- Explain the procedure to the patient to avoid surprises and difficulties while intubating
- Check medications. Some drugs may need to be avoided several days prior to the study
- Obtain patient history and complaints: symptoms, related test results, heart disease or asthma, allergy list
- Verify signed informed consent (if applicable for the institution).

Procedure

1 Soak solid state catheters in warm water for 1 h prior to the procedure to minimize catheter drift. This may optionally also be done for water-perfused catheters to make them softer and more comfortable for intubation
2 Have the patient sit upright
3 Let the patient inhale briskly through each nostril to find out which nostril is more open. Intubation should be performed through the nostril that is less obstructed
4 Test the gag reflex by touching the uvula or oropharynx. The risk for pulmonary aspiration is increased in patients who are unable to gag
5 Anesthetize patient's nare (e.g. Lidocaine spray or gel). Be aware that some patients may not want local anesthetics (LA) or may have had an allergic response on a previous occasion, so always ask the patient if they would like LA or not
6 Wait a few minutes for the effect of the anesthetics
7 Apply lubricating gel (e.g. Lidocaine gel) to the tip of the catheters
8 Gently insert the catheter straight back into the nose
9 When you feel the catheter slip into the nasopharynx, have the patient bring his/her *head forward* so that the chin touches the chest ("chin tuck"). Tilting the head forward encourages tracheal closure and passage of the catheter into the esophagus rather than the trachea
10 Ask the patient to breathe normally and to *swallow* while the catheter is being introduced into the nasopharynx. To make it easier to swallow the catheter, the patient may drink sips of water from a straw, while still sitting upright with the chin touching the chest
11 *Be aware* that the catheter should enter the esophagus easily and without coughing problems. Coughing may indicate that the catheter is misplaced (i.e. it may have slipped into the larynx). If the LES is hypertonic and shows poor relaxations to swallows there may be a problem in passing the catheter into the stomach. The catheter may curl around in the distal esophagus. In this case partially remove the catheter and slowly pass it down to the stomach again. If the entry is still impossible a guidewire may be introduced through the central lumen of a water-perfused catheter and the catheter may be advanced to the stomach under fluoroscopic guidance

12 Advance the catheter to its desired depth of insertion

13 Tape the catheter securely to the nose or cheek

14 Monitor patient's vital signs since nasogastric intubation and anxiety may result in the patient having vasovagal or fainting attacks

15 Allow the patient to acclimate to the catheter before commencing the study.

chapter 7

8 Clinical Procedures

8.1 Lower esophageal sphincter identification

The lower esophageal sphincter (LES) is the physiologic sphincter that separates the esophagus from the stomach. It is a high pressure zone with the purpose of limiting reflux of gastric contents to the esophagus.

The esophagus, together with the LES, passes down through the diaphragm to the stomach. During inspiration, downwards movement of the diaphragm generates a negative pressure change in the thoracic compartment (above the diaphragm), whereas a positive pressure change is seen in the abdominal compartment (below the diaphragm) due to compression of abdominal contents by the diaphragm (Fig. 8.1).

This phenomenon is used to orient the location of LES and to determine the intraabdominal and thoracic part of the LES (Fig. 8.2). When performing manometry the positive or negative direction of respiratory waves provides indication of the relative position of the pressure sensors (Fig. 8.3).

LES identification is important for accurate placement of catheters for 24-h pH-metry, bile reflux recordings, and motility recordings in the esophagus.

The location of the LES can be determined by:
- manometry—the best technique for accurate identification of LES
- built-in LES identifier (for pH-metry)
- pH step up (for pH-metry)
- fluoroscopy (will not identify the LES, but the site where the LES is most commonly located).

Manometry
EQUIPMENT
- Water-perfused or solid state catheter
- If using water-perfused catheter:
  (a) pneumohydraulic capillary infusion system

135

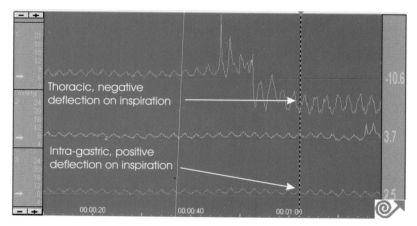

Figure 8.1 The proximal channel positioned above the diaphragm shows a *decrease* in pressure with each inspiration, whereas the distal channels positioned below the diaphragm show an *increase* in pressure with each inspiration.

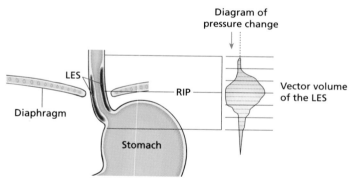

Figure 8.2 LES passing through the diaphragm. The pressure profile of the LES is shown by the vector volume of the LES.

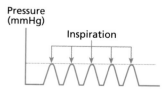

Figure 8.3 Quiet pressure change in stomach due to respiration. During inspiration there is a rise in pressure.

(b) tank of nitrogen

(c) sterile de-gassed distilled water

(d) pressure transducers and cables

- Multichannel recording system, e.g. Polygraf
- Computer, printer, analysis software program
- Accessories for nasal intubation.

PROCEDURE

1 Calibrate the equipment according to user's manual

2 Nasal intubation (see Section 7.6)

3 Position all channels (ports or sensors) which will record lower esophageal sphincter pressure (LESP) in the stomach

4 If the channels are indeed in the stomach, low-amplitude fluctuations should occur during respiration. During *inspiration*, there is a *rise* in pressure

5 Allow the patient to take a few deep breaths to confirm a positive deflection on inspiration. This verifies that the catheter channels are in the stomach. If the catheter is not positioned correctly partially remove it and slowly pass it down the stomach again (Fig. 8.4)

6 Set the gastric baseline, i.e. establish a reference baseline (a zero-value) at the average pressure in the stomach. The baseline is set either at the base of the respiration-associated waveform (the end-expiratory pressure), or in the middle of the waveform (the mid-respiratory pressure)

7 Perform a station or step pull through (SPT) of the LES by slowly pulling the catheter orad, in 0.5 or 1.0 cm increments, so that each channel will move through the LES. Each position should be maintained for at least 10 respiratory excursions

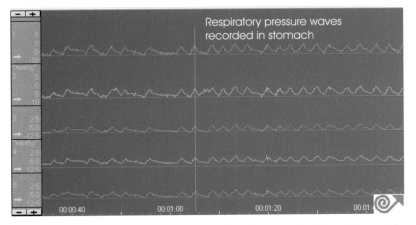

Respiratory pressure waves recorded in stomach

00:00:40   00:01:00   00:01:20   00:01

Figure 8.4 Motility recording with all channels in the stomach. The positions of the channels are identified by looking at the positive deflection on inspiration. Cursor positioned at the end-inspiratory point of respiration.

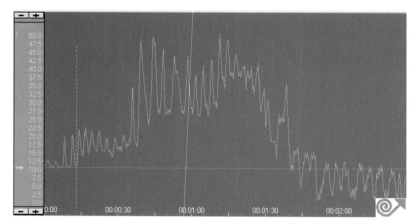

Figure 8.5 Station pull through of the LES. The red horizontal line is positioned at the end expiratory gastric baseline. The cursor shows the beginning of the LES where the pressure rises above the gastric end-expiratory baseline.

8 When the proximal recording site approaches the LES, the LES respiratory excursions will first increase as the sensor approaches the diaphragmatic crura. On entering the LES the basal tone will increase, this is the high pressure zone (Fig. 8.5). The distance in centimeters from the nares to the recording site is noted (note the markings on the catheter)

9 When the catheter channel is in the zone of high pressure, LES relaxation may be studied. Swallowing may accomplish a return to gastric baseline. If dry swallows do not accomplish this, try wet swallows (5–10 ml of room temperature water is gently squirted into the patient's mouth with a syringe). The LES relaxation verifies that the sensor is in the LES

10 As long as the LES is located below the diaphragm in the abdominal region, phasic pressure fluctuations during inspiration are positive. Once the channel traverses the diaphragm and enters the thoracic part of the LES, *inspiration* results in *negative pressure change*.

The respiratory inversion point (RIP) refers to that location where the pressure fluctuations related to inspiration change from positive to negative. Precisely at the RIP a biphasic respiratory fluctuation is often seen. The term pressure inversion point (PIP) may be used instead of RIP (Fig. 8.6)

11 When the proximal recording site leaves the LES and reaches the esophagus, basal pressure falls below the gastric baseline pressure (the intraesophageal pressure). The location at which this drop in pressure occurs marks the proximal end (upper border) of the LES. The distance in centimeters from the nares to this point is noted (Figs 8.7 & 8.8).

chapter 8

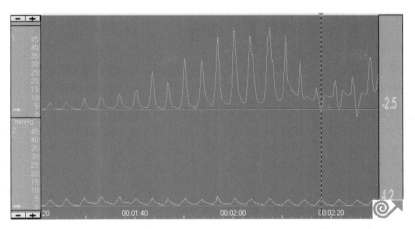

Figure 8.6 The cursor shows the respiratory inversion point (RIP). At this point the respiratory wave changes from a positive deflection with inspiration to a negative deflection.

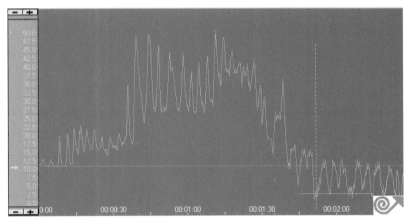

Figure 8.7 Station pull through of the LES. The cursor shows the position where the channel leaves the LES and enters the esophagus. The yellow horizontal line is positioned at the end-inspiratory esophageal baseline. Please observe the lower esophageal baseline compared to the intragastric baseline.

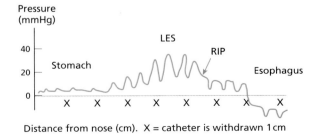

Distance from nose (cm). X = catheter is withdrawn 1 cm

Figure 8.8 Gastric, LES, and esophageal pressures as seen on a station pull through manometry study.

The built-in LES identifier

Some recorders for ambulatory 24-h pH-metry incorporate a built-in LES identifier to facilitate accurate placement of the pH catheter.

The system consists of three parts: (i) the unit with the built-in pressure sensor; (ii) an external pressure dome with an intravenous (IV) bag pressurized with a regular pressure cuff; and (iii) the pH catheters with a built-in pressure port.

The pressure changes are displayed on the recorder. The advantage of this system is that the patient only has to be intubated once. There is no need for additional intubation with a manometric catheter prior to pH-metry to determine LES location. However, this method is not as accurate as traditional manometry. The upper border of the LES may be difficult to define, but the RIP, however, is easily found.

EQUIPMENT (Fig. 8.9)
- Ambulatory 24-h pH-metry equipment
- Disposable or multiuse pH catheter with built-in pressure port for LES identification
- Pressure transducer
- Cable to connect pressure transducer with pH-metry equipment
- Pressure cuff
- Bag of sterile water in the cuff
- Micro drip set connected between the bag of sterile water and the pressure transducer
- Accessories for nasal intubation (see Chapter 7).

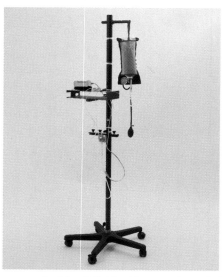

Figure 8.9 Equipment required for LES identification: the ambulatory pH recorder (Synectics Digitrapper Mk III); IV stand; bag of sterile water in pressure cuff; pH catheter with infusion channel.

PROCEDURE

1 Calibrate the pH electrode according to user's manual
2 Connect the transducer to the connector of the ambulatory 24-h pH-metry equipment
3 Connect the perfusion system
4 Inflate the cuff to a pressure of 300 mmHg to ensure a steady flow rate of 0.5 ml/min
5 Intubate the catheter through the patient's nose. Position the tip of the catheter 55 or 60 cm from the nose (see Chapter 7)
6 Place the patient in supine position
7 The menu on the pH recorder will display both pH values and a pressure bar (e.g. Synectics Digitrapper)
8 The pressure is zeroed when the pressure channel is positioned in the stomach
9 Gastric location is confirmed by asking the patient to take a slow deep breath. This should produce a positive pressure change (pressure bar moves to the right) (Fig. 8.10)

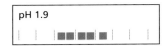

Figure 8.10 Intragastric positive pressure change with inspiration.

10 An SPT is then performed—withdraw the catheter in 0.5–1 cm steps, pausing at each step for 3–5 breaths
11 Ignore pressure changes in relation to swallows
12 As the LES is entered, the pressure variations become more prominent (Fig. 8.11)

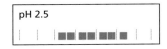

Figure 8.11 Range for LES pressure variations in the abdominal region.

13 At the RIP, the pressure becomes negative on inspiration (the bar moves to the left) (Fig. 8.12)

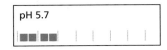

Figure 8.12 Range for LES pressure in the thoracic region. Pressure decreases with each inspiration.

14 On leaving the LES, pressure decreases below the gastric baseline and only minimal respiratory variations are seen. This is the upper border of the LES (Fig. 8.13).

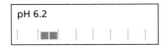

pH 6.2

Figure 8.13 Range for esophageal pressure variations. Negative with inspiration, but minimal respiratory variations.

Remember that the pressure recording port is located 5 cm above the tip of the pH electrode. To place the pH sensor 5 cm above the LES upper border, the pressure recording port should be withdrawn 10 cm above the upper border of the LES.

pH pull through "step-up"

In this technique the pH electrode alone is placed in the stomach and then withdrawn across the LES into the esophagus. The pH value is continuously observed on the display as the electrode is withdrawn. When the electrode enters the esophagus pH will rise: the location of this rise is considered to approximate the *lower* border of the LES. The tip of the pH electrode is then positioned 8 cm above this position (LES approx 3 cm (2–5 cm) + pH catheter 5 cm above the proximal LES border = 8 cm above the distal border of LES). This is not an accurate method and cannot be recommended.

Fluoroscopic guidance

With this method one is looking for the contour of the diaphragm or cardiac silhouette where the LES is most commonly located. It is not possible to visualize the LES itself with fluoroscopy. If the LES is displaced from its normal position in relation to the diaphragm, this will not be recognized using this method. This method is prone to considerable error and therefore cannot be recommended.

EQUIPMENT
• Catheter which can be visualized during fluoroscopy
• Fluoroscopy equipment
• Accessories for nasal intubation (see Chapter 7).

PROCEDURE
1 Nasal intubation (see Chapter 7)
2 Under fluoroscopic guidance withdraw the catheter from the stomach until it is located 5 cm proximal to the diaphragm or the inferior border of the cardiac silhouette.

chapter 8

8.2 24-h pH-metry
Indications
ESOPHAGEAL pH-METRY
- In patients with typical symptoms suggesting gastroesophageal reflux disease (GERD) without endoscopic esophagitis
- In patients with atypical symptoms (otorhinolaryngeal pathologies, non-cardiac chest pain, pulmonary problems)
- Pre- and postoperative evaluation of antireflux surgery

GASTRIC PH-METRY
- Titration of antireflux drugs
- In patients who have failed medical therapy for GERD.

Contraindications
- See contraindications for nasal intubation (see Chapter 7).

Equipment (Fig. 8.14)
- Battery powered ambulatory pH recorder
- pH catheter—antimony, ion-sensitive field effect transistor (ISFET) or glass electrode
- Buffer solution (pH 7.0 and 1.0)
- Analysis software
- Computer
- Printer
- Calibration stand
- Battery (9 V)

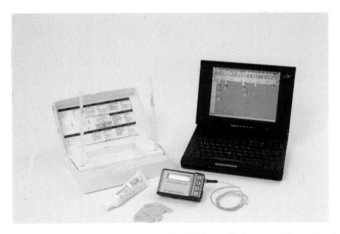

Figure 8.14 The Synectics Digitrapper Mk III for ambulatory pH monitoring and computer analysis software (Synectics PW EsopHogram Reflux Analysis Module). The photo also shows disposable accessories such as buffer solution, pHix strips (for attaching the catheter) and reference electrode gel.

143

- Accessories;
  (a) lubricating gel
  (b) anesthetic gel
  (c) electrode gel
  (d) cotton-tip applicators
  (e) tape
  (f) emesis basin
  (g) non-sterile gloves.

Before the study

- The patient should not ingest solids or liquids for at least 6 h prior to the pH study in order to minimize the risk of vomiting or aspiration, and to prevent buffering of gastric contents by food
- Discontinue all antacids 24 h prior to study. Proton pump inhibitors (e.g. omeprazole) should be discontinued 7 days prior to the study. All other medications known to interfere with gastric function or acid secretion should be discontinued 48 h prior to the study
- Assess patient information:
  (a) medical history
  (b) symptoms
  (c) medications
  (d) allergies
- Explain the procedure to the patient to promote cooperation and increase comfort level
- Verify signed informed consent (if applicable for the institution).

During the study

Activities
- Most major laboratory centers recommend the patient to continue his/her normal activities to get a more physiologic exam
- If patient is part of a controlled trial the laboratory centers standardize the exams giving instructions on meals, activities and sleeping time. In the standardized protocol the patient is recommended
  (a) to maintain an upright position throughout the day, i.e. sitting, standing, or walking position
  (b) lie down at night only to sleep
  (c) lay flat at night during sleep—one pillow only
- No baths or showers while the equipment is attached
- Handle the unit with care.

Sleep and posture
It is important to record periods of lying down and sleeping whether or not they occur at the same time.

Diet
- Most major laboratory centers allow the patient to continue his/her usual diet (sometimes prohibition only of acidic foods, carbonated, acidic and alcoholic drinks)
- No acid-inhibiting medications, no laxatives, antacids, aspirins, or non-steroidals should be taken during the test period
- Smoking is not permitted in most centers. If it is, remember that the patient has to note this in his/her diary.

Event buttons
If pH recorder has event buttons on its display, instruct the patient on how to operate these buttons. The buttons on the pH recorder are used to mark different periods and events. Examples of icons are given below:

 Chest discomfort/pain—heart burn

 Meals/eating

 Recumbent/sleep

 Used to mark other symptoms such as belch, hiccup, vomit, cough, and eventual periods when patient smokes.

Diary (Fig. 8.15)
Instruct the patient to keep a diary during the study to record meals, sleep, and symptoms noting their time of occurrence using the time displayed on the pH recorder. The patient should also specifically note any intake of acidic food—since this otherwise may be misinterpreted as reflux.

Procedure
1 Calibrate the equipment according to the user's manual
2 Anesthetize the nares (e.g. Lidocaine spray)
3 Insert pH catheter via the nares (see Chapter 7)
4 Pass the pH catheter into the stomach. The pH recorder will then display an acidic pH which verifies that the pH sensor is in the stomach. Withdraw the pH electrode slowly and place the sensor at the appropriate level. For a standard pH study, this point is 5 cm above the *upper* limit of the LES. The LES location should have been established either by reference to a prior manometric study, or by using the LES identifier in the pH recorder. In patients with combined esophageal and gastric pH monitoring, the optimal position of the gastric pH probe is 5 cm below the lower border of the esophageal sphincter
5 Fix the pH electrode in place by taping it to the nose and cheek. Tape it to the lower part of the neck after looping it over the ear (Fig. 8.16)

PATIENT DIARY

Name: _____   Date: _____

Start time: _____   End time: _____

Start time	End time	Meal 🍴	Reclining 🛏	Heart burn ♥	Chest pain	Belch	Regurg-itation	Other	Medication
Example:									
8:00									*Omeprazole*
12:45	13:30	X							
14:00				X					
22:00	06:00		X						

Comments:

Figure 8.15 Example of patient diary during the pH study period.

6 If a catheter with external reference is used, apply contact gel on the reference electrode, and then apply the electrode to the patient. Attach the reference in a location where it is less likely to be disturbed by the patient's movements, e.g. to the skin of the chest. Shave hair from the area and swab with alcohol to ensure good skin contact with the electrode

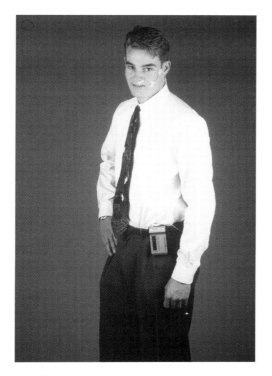

Figure 8.16 Patient with pH catheter *in situ*.

7 Attach the catheter to the pH recorder. Make sure the recorder is switched on and the pH value at the onset of the recording is accurate and is marked on the diary card prior to the patient leaving the department
8 Start the study and send patient home with diary, and instruction sheet
9 Have patient return to the laboratory on the next day. Stop the 24-h study
10 Disconnect the catheter from the pH recorder
11 Remove the catheter from the patient.

After the study

- If a reusable catheter has been used, remove organic debris by wiping and washing the catheter, then disinfect the catheter according hospital regulations and catheter manufacturer's instructions (e.g. after cleaning soak catheter for 20–30 min in glutaraldehyde (Cidex))
- Download the recording into the pH analysis software on a computer (Fig. 8.17) according to the software manufacturer's instructions
- The patient can resume his/her normal activities and diet, and recommence any discontinued medications.

147

chapter 8

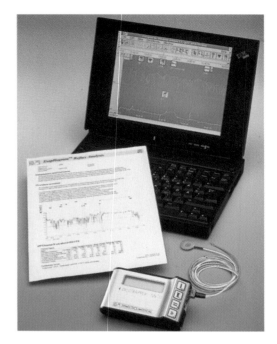

Figure 8.17 24-h pH study summary report.

Interpretations

With ambulatory esophageal pH monitoring one can detect the presence of gastroesophageal acid reflux (Fig. 8.18) and quantitate the actual time that the esophagus is exposed to acid gastric juice. One may categorize the reflux

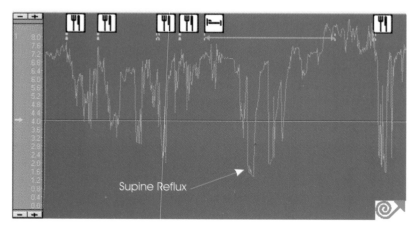

Figure 8.18 Tracing showing GERD. The patient presented with heartburn. 24-h pH-monitoring revealed an increased reflux pattern with reflux index/fraction time of 12%. In addition, frequent supine refluxes are shown.

in terms of upright, supine, or postprandial reflux. The test helps to correlate gastroesophageal reflux with symptoms and to discriminate between physiologic and pathologic reflux.

Several parameters may be considered in diagnosis of pathologic gastroesophageal reflux:

- the percentage of time pH is less than 4 (reflux index/fraction time)—this is the most valuable discriminator between physiologic and pathologic reflux. Many studies in normal populations suggest an upper limit of normal of 4.5–7% of total recording time with pH less than 4
- number of reflux episodes (below pH 4) lasting longer than 5 min during a 24-h study. This indicates the severity of the problem
- the longest reflux episode
- the relationship of reflux to eating, position, sleeping, activity, and symptoms.

DeMeester and Johnson scoring (Table 8.1)
The DeMeester and Johnson scoring incorporates several of these parameters. It measures the esophageal exposure to pH levels below pH 4 both by day and night. The score is composed of six parameters used to calculate the degree to which the patient's reflux pattern differs from the norm.

Table 8.1 DeMeester and Johnson scoring system.

24 h component	Mean ± SD	Normal value	Score
% time < pH 4 total	1.5 ± 1.4	<4.2	3.0
% time < pH 4 upright	2.3 ± 2.0	<6.3	2.98
% time < pH 4 supine	0.3 ± 0.5	<1.2	3.06
No reflux episodes < pH 4	20.6 ± 14.8	<50	2.99
No of episodes > 5 min	0.6 ± 1.3	3 or less	2.93
Longest episode (min)	3.9 ± 2.7	<9.2	3.0
Total score			17.96

The symptom index
The proportion of reflux episodes that correspond to an indicated symptom event is expressed as the symptom index. The formula is as follows:

$$\frac{\text{Number of symptoms when pH} <4}{\text{Total number of symptoms}} \times 100$$

A correlation of 50% or more has been suggested as being clinically significant.

The symptom association probability calculation
This is a statistical attempt to define the correlation between intermittent, atypical symptoms (especially chest pain) and reflux. This method statistically compares esophageal pH data temporally related to symptoms with pH data recorded during symptom-free episodes.

Pitfalls

- Care needs to be taken in the accurate placement of the electrodes in the esophagus
- If catheters with an external reference are used, it is important to prepare the skin properly, correctly attach the reference electrode (so it does not come loose during the study), and use the correct electrode gel. Displacement of external reference electrodes causes signal artifacts (unpredictable, rapidly changing pH)
- To obtain an adequate pH study, it is important to use fresh buffer solutions to calibrate the catheter. If the study is performed with antimony catheters remember that special buffers have to be used (without phosphate).

8.3 24-h bile study

Indications

This technique remains investigational. Clinical research studies may explore the use of this technology in the following situations:

- in patients with symptoms (including atypical symptoms) of gastro-esophageal reflux
- as a part of evaluation in patients with complications of gastroesophageal reflux such as:
  (a) Barrett's esophagus
  (b) strictures
  (c) ulceration of the esophagus
- in patients that have failed medical therapy for acid reflux
- in patients with poor response to medical treatment of reflux esophagitis
- in postgastrectomized patients with reflux symptoms
- pre- and postoperative evaluation of antireflux surgery.

Contraindications

- See contraindications for nasal intubation (see Chapter 7).

Equipment (Fig. 8.19)

- Ambulatory spectrophotometer
- Fiberoptic probe
- IBM-compatible computer
- Analysis software program
- Accessories:
  (a) lubricating gel
  (b) anesthetic gel

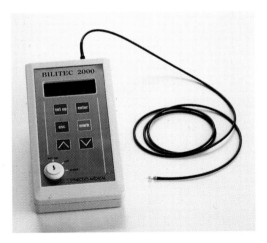

Figure 8.19 Synectics Bilitec for 24-h bile studies.

8

chapter

(c) cotton-tip applicators

(d) tape

(e) emesis basin

(f) non-sterile gloves.

Before the study

- The patient should not ingest solids or liquids for at least 6 h prior to the bile study to decrease the risk of vomiting, aspiration, and if pH-metry is to be performed simultaneously, to prevent buffering of gastric contents
- Discontinue all antacids 24 h prior to the study. Proton pump inhibitors (e.g. omeprazole) should be discontinued 7 days prior to the study. All other medications known to interfere with gastric function or acid secretion should be discontinued 48 h prior to the study
- Assess patient information:
  (a) medical history
  (b) symptoms
  (c) medications
  (d) allergies
- Explain the procedure to the patient in order to increase cooperation and comfort level
- Verify signed informed consent (if applicable for the institution).

During the study

Activities

- Some laboratory centers standardize the investigations, giving instructions on meals, activities, and time of sleeping. Other centers recommend that the patient continues his/her normal activities to get a more physiologic examination
- In standardized settings the patient is recommended
  (a) to maintain the upright position throughout the day—sitting, standing, or walking position
  (b) lie down only at night to sleep
  (c) lay flat at night during sleep—one pillow only
- No baths or showers as long as the equipment is attached
- Handle the unit with care.

Diet

- Food with a light absorbency similar to bilirubin should be avoided since it will interfere with bile reflux measurements
- Some centers only allow patients to have Nutridrink (e.g. a standardized liquid meal—banana flavor) during the 24-h study. Other centers give a list of food that may be eaten and a list with some foods that must be avoided
- Foods should be finely minced to avoid solid food aggregation on the tip of the probe

- No acid antisecretory medications, laxatives, antacids, aspirins, or non-steroidals should be taken during the test
- Smoking is not allowed in most centers.

Event button and diary
Instruct the patient on how to operate the event button on the recorder during the study. Also instruct the patient to keep a diary during the study, including notations and times.

Procedure

1 Calibrate the equipment according to the user's manual
2 Anesthetize the nares with local anesthetic spray (e.g. Lidocaine)
3 Put some lubricating gel on the tip of the probe for easier intubation
4 With the patient in the erect position, insert the probe into the nare (see Chapter 7)
5 The sensor tip is placed 5 cm above the upper border of the LES. To measure bile reflux into the stomach placement is 5–10 cm below the LES. For LES identification, see Chapter 7
6 Fix the probe in place by taping it to the nose and cheek. Tape it to the lower part of the neck after looping it over the ear
7 Connect the probe to the equipment and start the recording
8 Send patient home, with instructions regarding diet, activity, and of keeping a diary
9 Have patient return to lab the next day. Stop the recording
10 Remove the probe.

After the study

- The patient can resume his/her normal activities and diet and recommence any discontinued medications
- Disinfect the probe in glutaraldehyde (Cidex or similar solution) for 30 min. *Never* place the end of the probe that is connected to the unit in the cleaning solution. Gently dry the probe tip extremity with gauze. Replace the probe in its covering
- Transfer the data stored in the recorder to the personal computer. Process the data using a software program (e.g. Synectics EsopHogram reflux analysis module) (Fig. 8.20).

Pitfalls

- The recorder may underestimate bile reflux in an acidic medium (pH under 3.5) since bilirubin undergoes monomer to dimer isomerization in this environment and this results in a shift in the absorption wavelength from 453 to 400 nm
- A variety of substances in food may result in false-positive readings since the unit indiscriminately records any substances which absorb around 453 nm. Therefore, it is important to use a modified diet. Care should be

chapter 8

taken if long periods of bile reflux are recorded. This may be simply a contaminated detector or other artifact

- Be aware that the recorder measures reflux of bilirubin and not other duodenal components. In a few medical conditions (e.g. Gilbert's and Dubin–Johnson syndromes), there is a disproportionate secretion of bilirubin compared to other duodenal contents (especially bile acids).

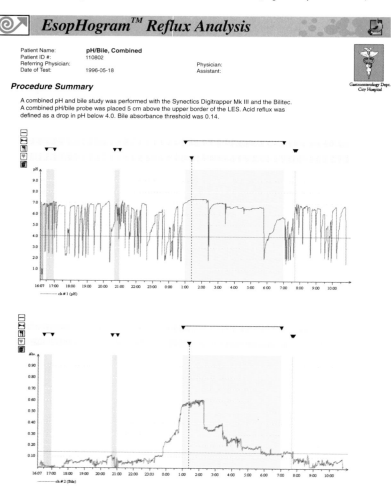

Figure 8.20 Two-page summary report of pH and bile recording (Synectics PW EsopHogram Reflux and Bile Analysis Module).

pH Channel 5 cm above the LES

Period Table

Item		Total	Upright	Supine	Meal	PostP
Duration of period	(HH:MM)	18:33	12:33	06:00	00:56	06:00
Number of acid refluxes	(#)	67	61	6	4	26
Number of long acid refluxes	(#)	5	4	1	0	1
Longest acid reflux	(min)	16	16	14	0	11
Total time pH below 4.00	(min)	116	99	17	1	43
Fraction time pH below 4.00	(%)	10.4	13.2	4.7	1.4	12.0
Symptom Index	(%)	n/a	n/a	n/a	n/a	n/a

DeMeester score
Total score = 32.6   DeMeester normals: <14.72 (95th percentile)

Bile Channel 5 cm above the LES

Period Table

Item		Total	Upright	Supine	Meal	PostP
Duration of period	(HH:MM)	18:33	12:33	06:00	00:56	06:00
Number of bile refluxes	(#)	54	25	30	4	6
Number of long bile refluxes	(#)	5	3	3	0	0
Longest bile reflux	(min)	360	73	287	3	1
Total time abs above 0.14	(min)	420	110	309	3	2
Fraction time abs above 0.14	(%)	37.7	14.7	85.9	5.8	0.5

3D-Graph - pH/Bile Absorbency - Total

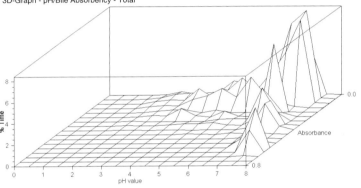

Frequency Distribution Graph - Total

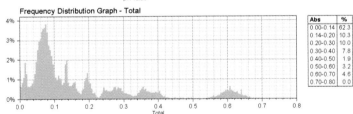

Abs	%
0.00-0.14	62.3
0.14-0.20	10.3
0.20-0.30	10.0
0.30-0.40	7.8
0.40-0.50	1.9
0.50-0.60	3.2
0.60-0.70	4.6
0.70-0.80	0.0

Signature:_____

PW - version 1.11 EsopHogram - version 1.0B4
Copyright © 1995-96, Synectics Medical AB

Date of test: 1996-05-18
pH/bile, Combined
110802

Figure 8.20 *Continued.*

8

chapter

8.4 Stationary esophageal manometry

Indications
- Evaluation of esophageal motility disorders:
  - (a) primary esophageal motility disorders (achalasia, nutcracker esophagus, diffuse esophageal spasm, hypertensive LES)
  - (b) nonspecific esophageal motility disorders
  - (c) secondary esophageal motility disorders—scleroderma, diabetes mellitus, chronic idiopathic intestinal pseudoobstruction (CIIP)
- Determination of LES prior to pH-metry (see Section 8.1)
- Preoperatively to exclude esophageal motility disorders if antireflux surgery is considered
- Dysphagia.

Contraindications
- See contraindications for nasal intubation (see Section 7.2).

Equipment (Fig. 8.21)
- Catheter
  - (a) water-perfused multilumen catheter. Hydraulic capillary infusion system. Normal standard infusion rate in adult esophageal manometry is 0.5 ml/min. The exact required infusion rate, however, depends on the diameter of the perfusion lumen—the rise rate (>300 mm/s) is

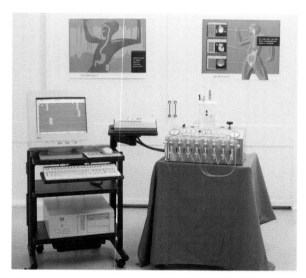

Figure 8.21 Equipment for stationary esophageal manometry. The photo shows the multichannel recording system Synectics PC Polygraf, the MUI perfusion pump and the computer with analysis software Synectics PW Esophageal Manometry Analysis Module.

the determining factor. Pressure transducers for each channel

or

(b) solid state catheter with built-in microtransducers
- Multichannel recording system (Polygraf)
- Device for monitoring swallows (optional)
- Respiratory transducer (optional—measures ribcage movements due to breathing)
- Personal computer with analysis software (e.g. esophageal manometry analysis module)
- Printer
- Accessories:
  (a) lubricating gel
  (b) anesthetic gel
  (c) cotton-tip applicators
  (d) tape
  (e) syringe 10–50 ml
  (f) emesis basin
  (g) nonsterile gloves
  (h) tissues
  (i) cup with straw.

Before the study (the patient)
- 48 h before the study, the patient should stop taking medications such as:
  (a) nitrates
  (b) calcium channel blockers
  (c) promotility agents
  (d) H_2-blockers
  (e) sedatives
  (f) analgesics
  (g) antidepressants
  (h) anticholinergics.

  If it is impossible to discontinue a medication affecting esophageal motility (e.g. nitrates, calcium channel blockers in cardiology patients, etc.) one must take this into account in the interpretation of results
- Patient should fast for at least 6 h prior to the study to decrease the risk of vomiting and aspiration
- Assess patient information:
  (a) medical history
  (b) symptoms
  (c) medications
  (d) allergies
- Verify signed informed consent (if applicable for the institution)
- Explain the procedure to the patient to increase patient cooperation and comfort level

• Instruct the patient to try not to talk, laugh, or swallow during the study unless asked to.

Before the study (the equipment)

• Calibrate the pressure channels according to user's manual
• Check that the manometric catheter is connected to the Polygraf so that the most proximal pressure channel appears at the top of the computer screen
• Prior to water-perfused manometry, carefully check that there are no air bubbles trapped in the pressure dome, capillaries, and tubing. The presence of air bubbles will significantly reduce response time and pressure readings. Carefully tap the domes and capillaries to release bubbles that might be trapped
• Optional testing prior to water-perfused manometry
(a) The occlusion test is a simple but useful way to check the performance of the system. Occlude the pressure port with a finger. Check the pressure rise time on the computer screen. Typically a system should be able to deliver more than 300 mmHg/s
(b) Check the performance of all channels by rapidly elevating the multi-lumen catheter from the mid level of the pressure dome to approximately 50 cm above the pressure dome. An identical rise-time and an equal maximum pressure should then be displayed in all channels.

Procedure

1 Lubricate the catheter and nasally intubate the patient, who should be sitting in an erect position (see Chapter 7)
2 Insert the catheter so that the channels which will record LESP are in the stomach just below the LES. Normally, at 60 cm all channels should be in the stomach
3 Position of patient:
(a) if water-perfused system is used, the patient is positioned in the supine position. The bed or transducer height should be adjusted so the transducers are placed at midaxillary level
(b) If a solid state catheter is used the patient does not need to be in a supine position
4 If a respiratory transducer is used, attach it to the lower edge of either side of the ribcage with tape or a fix strip. It measures movements of the ribcage with breathing. Have the patient breathe normally
5 Let the patient adjust to the catheter before starting the procedure (5–10 min). Verify tube placement by checking ability to talk and skin color.

MOTILITY STUDY

A complete motility study of the esophagus should include:

- LES study including LES relaxation study
- Esophageal body study
- Upper esophageal sphincter (UES) study.

LES study

There are five important factors to study:
- resting pressure—the high pressure zone (HPZ)
- overall length
- the length exposed to the positive pressure of the abdomen (abdominal length)
- the location of the upper (proximal) border of the LES—important for the placement of pH electrodes and other catheters
- adequate relaxation with wet swallow.

The procedure is as follows:

1 Verify that pressure channels are in the stomach by having the patient take a deep breath. Pressure should then rise in each of the channels located in the stomach. If any of the channels that should record the LES are not yet in the stomach, push the catheter down another 10 cm and verify location in the stomach (Fig. 8.22)

2 Set the gastric baseline, i.e. establish a reference baseline (a zero-value) at the average pressure in the stomach. The baseline is set either at the base of the respiration-associated waveform (the end-expiratory pressure) or in the middle of the waveform (the mid-respiratory pressure). Setting the gastric baseline makes it easy to detect changes in pressure in relation to this baseline. Record the baseline for at least 30 s

3 Perform the station and/or rapid pull throughs of the LES

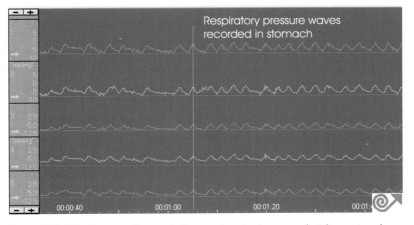

Figure 8.22 Motility recording with five openings in the stomach. The tracing shows that there is a positive pressure change with each inspiration in all five channels which verifies that these are in the stomach. The cursor is positioned at the end-inspiratory point of respiration.

4 *Station pull through.* Pull the catheter orad in 0.5–1 cm steps approximately every 15 s so that all the channels pass through the LES. Mark each catheter pull back (each new level) directly on the computer screen to keep track of the position of the catheter channels (distance from the nares). Some computers have a Windows interface where different icons are clicked on directly on the computer screen in order to illustrate different performances. Examples of icons are given below.

 Withdraw catheter icon: this is clicked each time the catheter is pulled back. It keeps track of the position of the catheter chan- -nels in the esophagus (distance from nares)

 Dry swallow icon: this figure is clicked on whenever the patient swallows

 The LES icon: the figure is clicked and positioned at the channel which is entering the LES

 The wet swallow icon: each time the patient is given water to swallow this icon should be clicked

5 Tell the patient not to swallow until specifically asked. If the patient swallows the LES relaxes and the resting tone is impossible to measure. Before moving the catheter again there has to be a pause for 15–20 s to allow the swallow to pass. Mark each accidental swallow directly on the computer screen (dry swallows)

6 When the proximal channel reaches the lower border of the LES there is sometimes an amplification of the respiration waves. A persistent rise in pressure exceeding 2 mmHg above the end-expiratory gastric baseline also indicates that the channel has entered the LES (the distal border of the LES). Mark the LES entry directly on the computer screen whenever a channel is entering the LES. If it is difficult to see the rise during the study it can be marked when the study is analyzed (Fig. 8.23)

7 While withdrawing the catheter the RIP (PIP) will be found. When the catheter channel passes through the diaphragm (from the abdominal side to the thoracic side) the pressure change due to respiration changes from a positive deflection with inspiration to a negative one (see Figs 8.24 & 8.25). The RIP refers to the location where this occurs. Since the LES is normally located where the esophagus passes through the diaphragm, the location of the RIP is normally within the LES. The RIP can be marked either directly on the computer screen while performing the study or afterwards when the study is analyzed

8 As the channel passes the proximal border of the LES, the pressure drops below the gastric baseline to the esophageal baseline. The overall length can then be defined as the distance in centimeters, from the first rise >2 mmHg above the gastric baseline to the fall to intraesophageal baseline

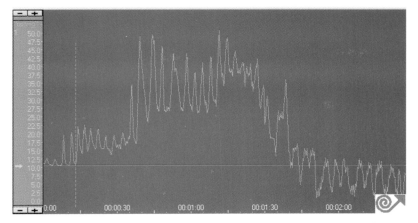

Figure 8.23 Station pull through of the LES. The persistent rise in pressure above the gastric baseline indicates that the channel has entered the LES. The red horizontal line is positioned at the end expiratory gastric baseline. The cursor shows the beginning of the LES.

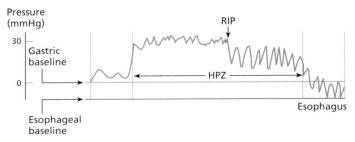

Figure 8.24 The HPZ seen when the catheter is withdrawn from the stomach to the esophagus.

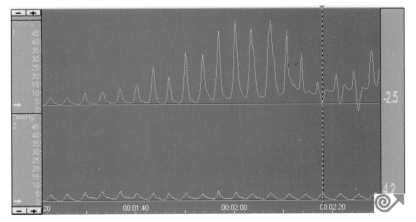

Figure 8.25 Station pull through of the LES. The respiratory inversion point (RIP) is found where the respiratory wave changes from a positive deflection with inspiration to a negative deflection. The cursor marks the RIP.

9 Repeat pull-throughs with the pressure channels that follow, to obtain adequate LES data

10 *An optional test*: with the catheter channel within the LES at various levels ask the patient to stop breathing on exhalation for a few seconds. A baseline pressure of the LES will then be recorded without respiratory artifacts. This baseline can be used for calculation of end-expiratory LES resting pressure

11 *Rapid pull through*: connect the catheter to an automatic puller which withdraws the catheter at a continuous speed of 0.5–1.0 cm/s, as respiration is suspended. The LES pressure rise and fall is identified in a similar way as with the LES slow pull through technique.

Data obtained by stationary (or rapid) pull through of the LES
- The distal and proximal border of the LES
- The overall length of the LES: the length from distal LES to proximal LES (normal value 2.4–5.5 cm)
- The abdominal length of the LES: the length from distal LES to RIP (normal value 0.8–5 cm) (Fig. 8.26)

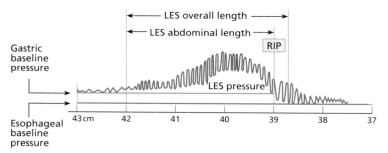

Figure 8.26 The overall and abdominal length of the LES can be calculated from the pull through manometric profile of the LES:

Overall length = location of distal LES − location of proximal LES
(e.g. 42 − 38.5 = 3.5 cm)
Abdominal length of LES = location of distal LES − location of RIP
(e.g. 42 − 39 = 3 cm)

- The LES pressure: the pressure (either end-expiratory or mid-respiratory) above the gastric baseline in the LES is called the resting pressure of the LES. The methods to obtain the resting pressure differ in terms of the location and the point in the respiratory cycle at which LES pressure is measured. The normals for LES pressure differ depending on what method is used. The four methods commonly used are as follows:

1 Maximum end-expiratory pressure (Fig. 8.27)
- Exclude sections with LES relaxations
- Use the end-expiratory intragastric baseline as the zero reference and identify the highest end-expiratory pressure in the LES. The channel

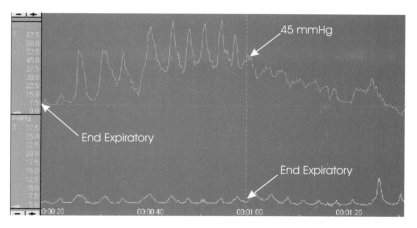

Figure 8.27 LES maximum end-expiratory pressure.

positioned in the stomach shows the slight pressure wave due to respiration. By placing a vertical cursor at the trough of the wave (end-expiratory
intragastric pressure) the maximum end-expiratory pressure of the LES will
easily be found (see Fig. 8.27)

- Take a mean value from several LES recordings.

2 Mean pressure over the HPZ (Fig. 8.28)

- Exclude sections with LES relaxations
- Use the mid-respiratory intragastric baseline as the zero reference and
  identify the HPZ of the LES. Calculate the mean (the average pressure)
  of the mid-respiratory LES pressures in the HPZ
- Take the mean value from several LES recordings
- Using this method, for example, the Castell Laboratory defines normal
  LES pressure as 14–34 mmHg at mid-respiration for water-perfused

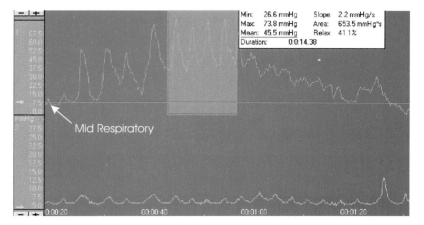

Figure 8.28 Mean pressure over the HPZ of the LES.

catheters. With the solid state circumferential transducer 17–35 mmHg is considered normal.

3 Mid-respiration pressure at the RIP (Fig. 8.29)
- Exclude sections with LES relaxation
- Identify the RIP by looking for the change in deflection from a positive pressure change with inspiration to negative. Use the mid-respiratory intragastric baseline as the zero reference and calculate the LES pressure (at mid-respiration) at the RIP
- Take a mean value from several LES recordings
- The DeMeester Laboratory, for example, uses this method with normal LES pressure at the RIP between 6 and 26 mmHg (water-perfused catheters).

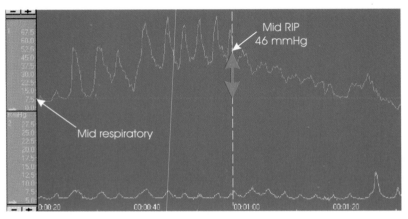

Figure 8.29 LES pressure at the RIP.

4 Mid-respiratory pressure (Fig. 8.30)
- Exclude sections with LES relaxations
- Use mid-respiratory intragastric baseline as zero reference and identify the HPZ. Calculate the mid-respiratory pressure of the HPZ
- Take a mean value from several LES recordings (Table 8.2).

The normal values are slightly different among laboratories, not only because of different measuring techniques, but also because of technical differences (type of catheter, perfusion pressure and rate, compliance of the system, sampling rate, etc.).

LES relaxation study

After the pull throughs of the sphincter have been performed continue with the LES relaxation study. Two important parameters need to be defined:
- coordination of LES relaxation to swallowing
- the degree of LES relaxation or the residual pressure on relaxation— defined as the pressure difference between gastric baseline and the lowest sustained pressure at LES relaxation.

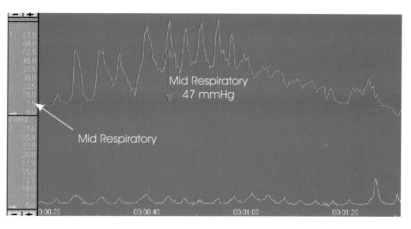

Figure 8.30 Mid-respiratory pressure.

The technique is as follows:

1 Place at least one channel in the stomach to show the gastric baseline, and one channel in the HPZ of the LES

Table 8.2 Normal values for LES pressures. Reproduced from Schuster, 1993 with the permission of Williams & Wilkins.

Infused manometry (mean of four orifices at 90)	Pressure (mmHg; mean ± SD)
RPT	29.0 ± 12.1
SPT	
end-inspiration	39.7 ± 13.2
mid-respiration	24.2 ± 10.1
end-expiration	15.2 ± 10.7
Solid-state circumferential ("sphincter") transducer	26.0 ± 9.4

2 Give the patient a series of wet swallows (e.g. ten) to assess the relaxation at the LES on swallowing (Fig. 8.31). Since the patient is normally in a supine position, the easiest way to give the water is by a 10–50 ml syringe. A 5–10 ml bolus of water at room temperature should be given each time. Mark each swallow directly on the computer screen. Wait for at least 20–30 s between each wet swallow:

(a) if there is complete relaxation of the LES, the pressure drops almost to the gastric baseline

(b) complete relaxation is defined as 90% relaxation (a residual pressure of less than 5 mmHg)

(c) per cent relaxation (Fig. 8.32):

$$\frac{\text{Resting} - \text{residual pressure}}{\text{Resting pressure}} \times 100 = \% \text{ relaxation}$$

(d) Residual pressure is the pressure between the gastric baseline and the lowest sustained 3-s interval of LES pressure.

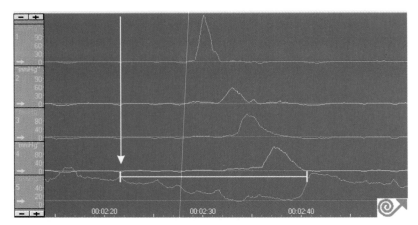

Figure 8.31 LES relaxation due to a swallow. The cursor marks the beginning of the pharyngeal spike which is also when the LES relaxation occurs. The horizontal white line shows the duration of the LES relaxation.

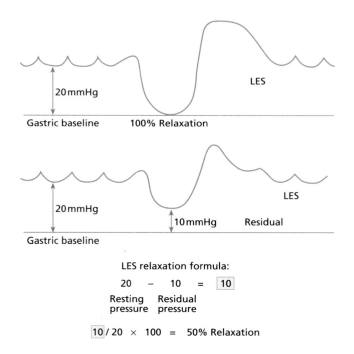

Figure 8.32 LES relaxation formula.

Esophageal body study

The esophageal body is studied in order to determine the strength and duration of the esophageal contractions. Four parameters should be evaluated:

- peristalsis: the sequential progression of the wave from which the propagation velocity is calculated
- amplitude of the contractions
- duration of the contractions
- the number of peaks per contraction.

The technique is as follows:

1 Position the distal channel 3 cm above the proximal border of LES. (When the distal channel is in the LES, the catheter can be pulled back slowly noting when the pressure drops to the esophageal baseline level. From there the catheter is pulled back another 3 cm)

2 Verify that all the channels are in the esophagus by having the patient inspire deeply and observing negative deflection in all pressure channels

3 Secure the catheter in place by gently taping it to the patient's nose

4 Have the patient perform 7–15 wet swallows 20–30 s apart. Give the patient a 5–10 ml bolus of room temperature water from a 10–50 ml syringe. Mark each swallow directly on the computer. There has to be at least 20–30 s between each wet swallow. If the patient swallows too frequently the contractile activity will be inhibited and may be misinterpreted as abnormal activity

5 Encourage the patient not to cough, talk, or swallow between the wet swallows

6 Unfasten catheter from the patient's nose and pull the catheter back another 7 cm (not necessary if it is a catheter with several (e.g. eight) channels since the proximal esophagus has then already been examined)

7 Tape the catheter to the patient's nose and repeat the wet swallow procedure. Perform a series of 10 wet swallows to examine the proximal esophagus. Mark each swallow directly on the computer screen.

Data obtained from the esophageal body function study

- Amplitude: the highest peak of contraction is measured from the baseline. 10 mmHg is considered to be the measurable threshold of contraction (Table 8.3). If the amplitude is greater than 180 mmHg, the contractions are considered to be hypertensive (nutcracker)
- Duration: measured from the major upstroke to the end of the wave
- Propagation rate/velocity is calculated as the time taken for a contraction wave to migrate a known distance. The distance between two pressure sensors is divided by the time delay between onset of the peristaltic wave in each channel
- Contractions may occur in peristaltic, simultaneous, interrupted, or dropped sequences (Figs 8.33–8.35). Multipeak contraction (see Fig. 8.33) is defined as a contraction with more than one peak. Each peak must

Table 8.3 Normal values for esophageal peristalsis (mmHg; mean ± SD). Reproduced from Schuster, 1993 with the permission of Williams & Wilkins.

Recording site (cm above LES)	Wet swallows	Dry swallows	P value
Amplitude (mmHg; mean ± SD)			
18	62 ± 29	44 ± 25	<0.001
13	70 ± 32	48 ± 27	<0.001
8	90 ± 41	63 ± 32	<0.001
3	109 ± 45	79 ± 33	<0.001
mean: 8/3	99 ± 40	71 ± 28	<0.001
Duration (s; mean ± SD)			
18	2.8 ± 0.8	2.6 ± 0.7	NS
13	3.5 ± 0.7	3.4 ± 0.6	NS
8	3.9 ± 0.9	3.8 ± 0.8	NS
3	4.0 ± 1.1	4.2 ± 0.8	NS
mean: 8/3	3.9 ± 0.9	4.1 ± 0.8	NS
Velocity (cm/s; mean ± SD)			
Proximal	3.0 ± 0.6	4.0 ± 0.4	<0.001
Distal	3.5 ± 0.9	4.0 ± 0.3	<0.001

NS, not significant.

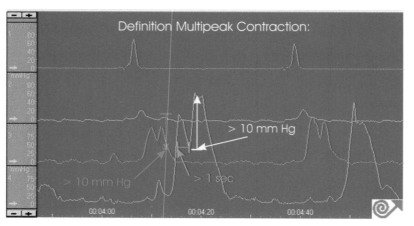

Figure 8.33 Definition of multipeak contractions.

satisfy the following criteria: (i) peak to trough interval longer than 1 s; (ii) peak to trough decline more than 10 mmHg; (iii) trough to peak amplitude greater than 10 mmHg (see Fig. 8.33).

UES study (Figs 8.36 & 8.37)
In order to acquire a complete esophageal motility study, the UES should also be studied. However, if oropharyngeal swallowing disorders are suspected, this study should be performed with a specially designed assembly and in conjunction with videofluoroscopy (see p. 188).

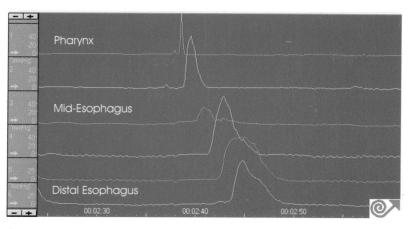

Figure 8.34 Normal esophageal peristalsis showing low contraction amplitude at the transition zone between striated and smooth muscle fibers in the esophagus.

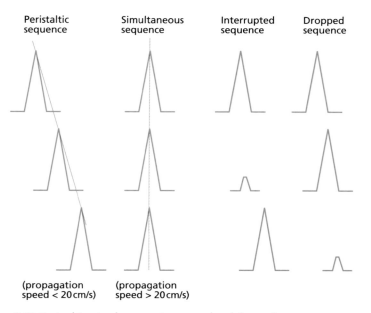

Figure 8.35 Peristaltic, simultaneous, interrupted and dropped sequence.

Three parameters may be examined:
- the resting pressure: the pressure above the esophageal baseline
- relaxation: the pressure drops to baseline with swallowing
- coordination between the pharyngeal peristalsis and cricopharyngeal (UES) relaxation.

The technique is as follows:
1 Slowly pull the catheter back in 1-cm steps every 10–15 s with breaks to assess UES relaxation

169

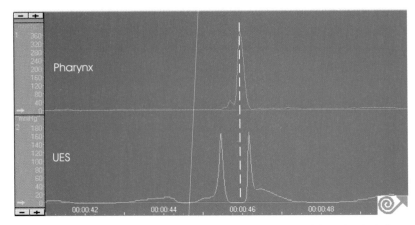

Figure 8.36 UES manometry with a solid state catheter in a healthy individual showing coordination of the pharyngeal contraction with UES relaxation. The cursor shows that the pharyngeal spike occurs simultaneous with the nadir of UES relaxation.

2 A pressure rise above the esophageal baseline marks that the proximal channel has reached the lower border of the UES. Mark the UES directly on the computer screen or afterwards when analyzing the study. Examples of icons used in an esophageal analysis program are given below:

 UES icon to click on the computer screen when channel enters the UES

 Wet swallow icon to click on when bolus of water is given the patient

3 A fall in pressure to pharyngeal pressure marks the upper border of the UES

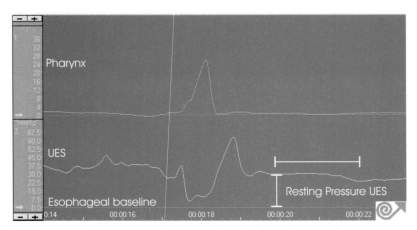

Figure 8.37 UES manometry with water-perfused catheter showing the resting pressure of the UES. The red horizontal line shows the esophageal baseline which is the zero reference line when calculating the mean resting pressure of the UES.

4 The highest resting pressure in the sphincter is defined as basal sphincter pressure. Due to asymmetry of the UES, this is normally 50–100 mmHg depending on direction of the pressure sensor, i.e. whether lateral or anterior/posterior

5 Continue the pull back of the catheter so that the second channel also enters the UES. One pressure channel is then located in the pharynx, one in the UES, and at least one in the esophagus

6 Perform a series of wet swallows to study UES relaxation and correlation of sphincter relaxation with pharyngeal contraction. Five milliliters water at room temperature is given to the patient. Each wet swallow is marked on the computer screen. Do a series of at least four swallows

7 Keep withdrawing the catheter 1 cm at a time until all channels have passed through the UES into the pharynx. The swallows can be repeated as each channel is located in the UES. If a water-perfused system is used, turn off the ports located in the pharynx to avoid the irritation in the pharynx

8 Remove the catheter and, if the respiratory and swallow transducer have been used, disconnect them from the patient.

After the study
- Obtain and document the patient's vital signs
- Instruct the patient that cold gargle may be used for minor throat irritation
- The patient can resume his/her normal activities and diet and restart any discontinued medication. Remember to report if the patient had not discontinued medication affecting esophageal motility
- Clean and disinfect the catheter according to hospital regulations and catheter manufacturer's instructions.

Stationary esophageal manometry with sleeve technique

Monitoring of the LES and UES sphincter pressure, in fact any sphincter pressure, poses some specific challenges to the clinician. Traditionally this has been done with a multilumen catheter with perfused side holes and an SPT technique.

The challenge of traditional LES manometry is due to a combination of the following factors.

Narrowness of the maximum pressure zone of the LES
Typically the area of the maximum pressure of the LES and UES is only a part of the actual HPZ. In an adult population this is less than 5 mm.

Mobility of the sphincter
The mobility of the UES and LES has been well documented and amounts to 1.5–2 cm in conjunction with a swallow.

Directional property of pressure sensors/ports
The directional properties of a water-perfused side hole or a directional

chapter 8

solid state sensor records only the pressure in very close relation to the actual pressure sensor or port.

Changes of resting pressure over time

It has been stated that the resting pressure of the LES varies with time. Suggested value varies typically from 10 to 35 mmHg.

The challenges of the mobility of the sphincters together with the directional pressure sensors and the narrow zone of maximal sphincter pressure makes it difficult to measure accurate sphincter responses relative to swallowing. This has led to the development of so-called "sleeve sensors" (e.g. Dentsleeve Pty Ltd).

The sleeve sensor consists of a concave molded bed, 6 cm long, to exceed the movements of the sphincter. The bed is covered with a thin silicone membrane where the water enters at the proximal end and perfuses freely through the distal part of the membrane. The sleeve with its long membrane then allows for a secure continuous recording with an anchored assembly and eliminates the need for repeated pull through. It may also be used to measure accurate sphincter pressure over time.

A typical assembly for stationary esophageal manometry is shown in Fig. 8.38 where a 6-cm long sleeve is used in combination with regular directional pressure ports.

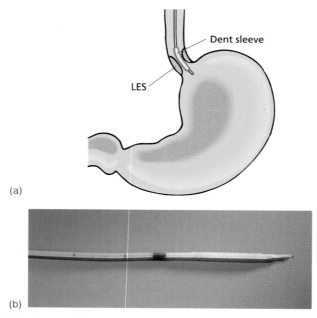

(a)

(b)

Figure 8.38 The Dent sleeve and its position during LES manometry. Eight-channel assembly: distal channel = intragastric; LES sleeve = 6 cm pressure sensor membrane; five directional pressure sensors for esophageal peristalsis with 3–5 cm spacing; pharyngeal sensor = perfused at very low rate 0.15 ml/min or perfused with air.

PROCEDURE WITH A SLEEVE SENSOR

LES and esophageal body study

1 Position at least three pressure channels in the stomach to verify placement (60 cm insertion depth)
2 Perform an SPT of LES with the directional pressure channels in order to determine the location of the LES
3 Position the center of the sleeve in the middle of the LES
4 Check pharyngeal channel for identifications of swallows
5 Perform 10 wet swallows with a 5 ml standardized bolus to obtain esophageal contractions and LES relaxations.

UES study

1 Withdraw catheter and perform an SPT of the UES with the directional channels to verify UES position
2 If a water-perfused catheter is used, close the excessive proximal ports of the catheter to avoid water-induced irritation and swallowing
3 Position the center of the sleeve in the UES
4 Record UES resting pressure with the sleeve
5 Perform five wet swallows with 5 ml room temperature water by syringe to obtain UES relaxation due to swallowing
6 Optional: give patient three swallows with 5, 10, and 20 ml room temperature water by a syringe to check swallow and relaxation as well as correlation of increase in intrabolus pressure with increase in given volume of water.

Optional procedure

In order to study secondary esophageal peristalsis the catheter can optionally be supplied with a balloon or air infusion port. The balloon distention or air infusion provocation test is used to provoke secondary peristalsis.

Interpretations

Achalasia

There is a characteristic manometry pattern for achalasia (Figs 8.39 & 8.40):

- absence of esophageal peristalsis
- elevated LES pressure—over 45 mmHg
- incomplete relaxation of the LES
- when the esophagus body is dilated there is an elevated intraesophageal baseline pressure.

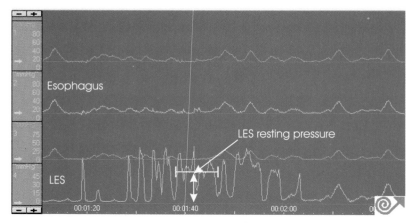

Figure 8.39 Patient with achalasia showing absence of peristalsis in the distal esophagus, high LES pressure and elevated esophageal baseline.

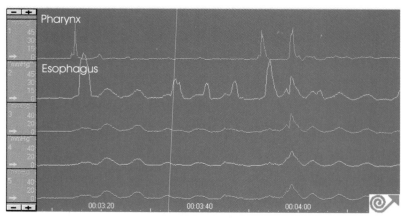

Figure 8.40 Patient with achalasia. There is peristaltic contractile activity in the pharynx and the proximal esophagus consisting of striated muscle fibers, but no peristalsis in the distal esophagus consisting of smooth muscle fibers. Tracings from the distal esophagus show a typical mirroring effect (identical tracings) which is a common phenomenon in achalasia.

Diffuse esophageal spasm

These are the common manometric abnormalities to verify the diagnosis of diffuse esophageal spasm (DES) (Figs 8.41 & 8.42):

- frequent simultaneous (nonperistaltic) contractions (more than 20–30% of wet swallows), separated by periods of normal peristalsis
- manometric abnormalities in DES are usually but not always confined to the distal two-thirds of the esophagus
- multiphasic waves (more than two peaks per wave)
- prolonged duration of contractions (more than 6 s)

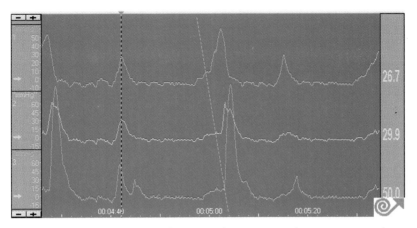

Figure 8.41 Patient with DES. The cursor shows one simultaneous wave and one peristaltic wave.

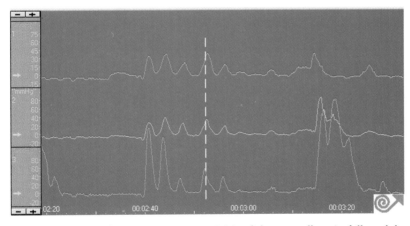

Figure 8.42 DES. The contraction wave initiated by a swallow is followed by multiple spontaneous simultaneous contractions of low amplitude. The cursor shows a simultaneous contraction.

- spontaneous contractions
- high-amplitude contractions (greater than 180 mmHg).

Nutcracker esophagus

These are the manometric abnormalities that have been proposed for nutcracker esophagus (Figs 8.43 & 8.44):

- high-amplitude peristaltic contractions above 180 mmHg. Contraction amplitudes can commonly exceed 300 mmHg in these patients
- contractions of prolonged duration and increased LES pressure may be present.

8

chapter

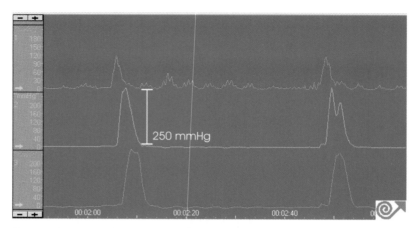

Figure 8.43 Nutcracker esophagus. The tracing shows high amplitude peristaltic esophageal contractions (>180 mmHg).

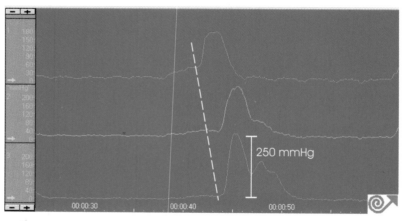

Figure 8.44 Nutcracker esophagus variant. The tracing shows multiple peaked waves that are peristaltic, high amplitude and of prolonged duration (in contrast to DES where these multiple peaked waves are often simultaneous).

Hypertensive LES

Hypertensive LES is considered by some as a primary esophageal motility disorder. Others dispute its existence as a separate entity. As in achalasia the LES pressure is elevated, but in contrast to achalasia esophageal peristalsis is normal.

Manometric criteria are as follows:
- elevated LES pressure—over 45 mmHg
- normal esophageal peristalsis (Fig. 8.45).

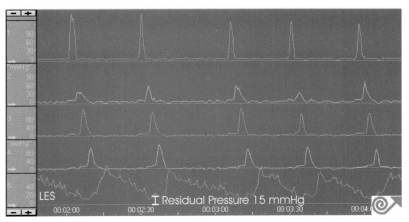

Figure 8.45 Hypertensive LES with incomplete relaxation (residual pressure 15 mmHg). Normal esophageal peristalsis is shown.

Nonspecific esophageal motor disorder
Each of these manometric findings may be included under the term non-specific esophageal motor disorder (NEMD) (Fig. 8.46):
- increased number of multipeaked or repetitive contractions
- contractions of prolonged duration
- nontransmitted contractions—interruption of peristaltic waves at various levels of the esophagus
- contractions of low amplitude
- isolated abnormal LES function.

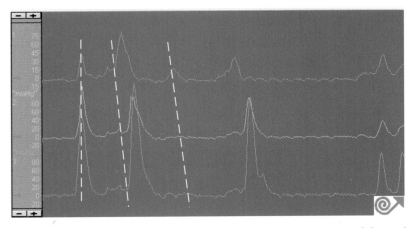

Figure 8.46 NEMD. A mixed picture with simultaneous, propagating, and dropped esophageal peristalsis.

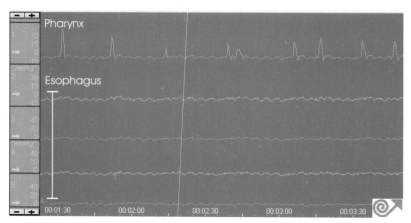

Figure 8.47 Tracing from a patient with scleroderma: absence of distal esophageal peristalsis, low esophageal baseline pressure.

Scleroderma

These are esophageal manometry patterns typical of scleroderma (Fig. 8.47):
- decreased LES pressure leading to gastroesophageal reflux (incompetent LES)
- weak or absent distal esophageal contractions and peristalsis
- normal upper esophageal contraction, peristalsis, and UES pressure
- normal LES relaxations.

Oropharyngeal swallowing disorders

While conventional manometry may detect abnormalities in the UES and pharynx the clinical interpretation of such findings must be mindful of the technical limitations of the technology.

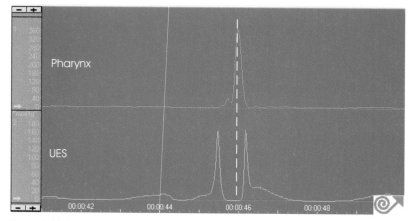

Figure 8.48 UES manometry in a healthy individual. The cursor shows that the pharyngeal spike occurs simultaneous with the nadir of UES relaxation.

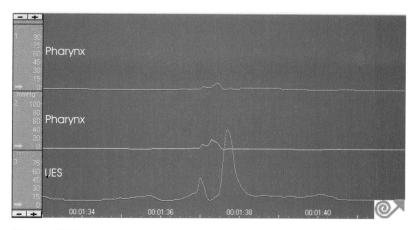

Figure 8.49 Patient with dysphagia showing poor pharyngeal contractions, but normal coordination with UES relaxation.

Motility abnormalities of the pharynx and UES which may result in dysphagia (Figs 8.48 & 8.49) are:
• weak pharyngeal contractions
• incomplete relaxation of UES
• uncoordinated pharyngeal contraction and UES relaxation.

A summary report of esophageal manometry is shown in Fig. 8.50.

Esophageal Manometry

Patient Name:	**Esophageal, Demonstration**		
Patient ID #:	620522-5682		
Referring Physician:	Yuen, K	Physician:	Johnsson, E
Date of Test:	1996-01-18	Assistant:	Roberts, B

Gastroenterology Dept.
Cay Hospital

Interpretation and Comments

Overall, peristalsis is sufficient but is sometimes disrupted. No evidence of non-specific disorders or spasm. Esophageal contractions and LES resting pressure are normal but border on being hypotensive.

Recommend a 24 hour pH study to determine if chest pain is related to reflux.

LES Station Analysis (Wet Swallows)

Location :	56.0 to 51.0 cm	<u>Normals</u>
Resting pressure :	14.0 mmHg	14.3 to 34.5 mmHg
Mean gastric baseline:	4.9 mmHg	
Residual pressure:	0.9 mmHg	less than 5.0 mmHg
Percent relaxation:	91.1%	greater than 90%

Schuster M, Castell J, Gideon RM, Castell DO; "Atlas of Gastrointestinal Motility in Health and Disease, Baltimore, Williams and Wilkins, 1993, pp 134-157.
Richter JE, Wu Wc, Johns DN, Blackwell JN, Nelson JL, Castell JA, Castell DO, Esophageal manometry in 95 healthy volunteers adult volunteers. Dig Dis Sci 1987; 32:583-592.

Esophageal Motility Analysis (Wet Swallows)

Total number of swallows :	9
Peristaltic normal :	55 %
Peristaltic hypertensive :	0 %
Peristaltic hypotensive :	0 %
Simultaneous or uncoordinated :	44 %

	Distal
Contractions :	22
Multipeaked (%) :	0
Mean amplitude (mmHg) :	45.0
Mean duration (sec) :	2.7
Peristaltic (%) :	62

Standard UES Analysis (Wet Swallows)

Location :	24.0 to 21.0 cm
Resting pressure :	51.0 mmHg
Residual pressure :	-4.8 mmHg
UES / pharynx coordination :	75 %

Tracing Clip-Outs

Example 1

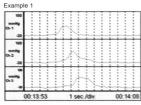

Example 2

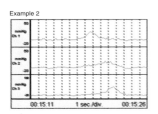

Signature : _____

Copyright © 1995-1996, Synectics Medical AB

PW - version 1.11
Esophageal Manometry - version 1.01

Figure 8.50 One-page summary report of esophageal manometry (Synectics PW EsopHageal Manometry Analysis Module).

8
chapter

8.5 Ambulatory esophageal manometry

The main use of 24-h ambulatory esophageal manometry is to correlate intermittent symptoms such as chest pain, dysphagia, and heartburn to motor abnormalities.

With ambulatory 24-h manometry, the number of esophageal contractions available for analysis increases. It provides, therefore, an opportunity to assess esophageal motor functions in combination with pH-metry in a variety of physiologic situations such as sleep, waking periods, and meal periods.

The diseases listed below may be missed due to the limited study time when performing stationary esophageal manometry, but found with 24-h ambulatory manometry.

Indications
Suspected diseases such as:
- DES
- nutcracker esophagus
- nonspecific esophageal motility disorders,

and symptoms such as:
- noncardiac chest pain
- intermittent dysphagia.

Contraindications
- See contraindications for nasal intubation (see Chapter 7).

Equipment
- Ambulatory data recorder—combined pH and motility recorder (Fig. 8.51)
- Solid state catheter. The standard catheter for ambulatory esophageal motility studies consists of three pressure transducers positioned 5 cm

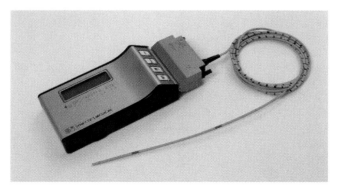

Figure 8.51 The ambulatory data recorder Synectics MicroDigitrapper with a solid state small bowel motility catheter.

apart and radially oriented at 120° intervals. If a combination of motility recording and pH-metry should be performed the catheter could be combined with one or two pH sensors, or a separate pH catheter (preferably antimony with internal reference or ISFET catheter) could be used together with the solid state pressure catheter. If LES data should be recorded, a sleeve catheter or a sphinctometer should be used

- Personal IBM-compatible computer with analysis software
- Printer
- Buffers for calibrating pH sensors
- Calibration chamber for pressure sensors
- Batteries (9 V alkaline batteries)
- Accessories:
  (a) lubricating gel
  (b) anesthesic gel
  (c) cotton-tip applicators
  (d) tape or pHix strips
  (e) syringe 10–50 cm^3
  (f) emesis basin
  (g) non-sterile gloves
  (h) tissues
  (i) cup with straw
  (j) gel for reference electrode (if external reference on pH catheter).

Before the study

- 48 h prior to the study, the patient should stop taking medications such as:
  (a) nitrates
  (b) calcium channel blockers
  (c) promotility agents
  (d) sedatives
  (e) analgesics
  (f) antidepressants
  (g) H$_2$-blockers
  (h) anticholinergics.
  If it is impossible to discontinue a medication affecting esophageal motility (e.g. nitrates, calcium channel blockers in cardiology patients, etc.) one must take this into account in interpretation
- Patient should stop taking antacids 24 h before the study. Proton pump inhibitors (e.g. omeprazole) should be stopped 7 days before the study
- Exceptions to discontinuation of medications are in some situations when it may be of interest to study patients while they are taking their medications
- Patient comes to the esophageal laboratory after an overnight fast to avoid aspiration (at least 6 h of fasting)
- Assess patient information:

(a) medical history.
(b) symptoms
(c) medications
(d) allergies
- Explain the procedure to the patient to increase patient cooperation and comfort level
- Verify signed informed consent (if applicable for the institution).

During the study

Activities
- Normal activities
- No baths or showers as long as the equipment is attached.

Diet
- Continue normal diet. Most centers have no diet restrictions since the recording should be as physiologic as possible
- In more standardized settings the patient is given instructions such as:
  (a) all meals must be eaten at one sitting within a 30-min period and they should be at least 4 h apart. This is to avoid long periods where swallowing is a part of food ingestion
  (b) no chewing gum
  (c) patient should not eat/drink any carbonated beverage, tea, coffee, alcohol, fruit juices, tomatoes, or candy which increases gastroesophageal reflux and esophageal acidity
- No acid antisecretory medications, laxatives, antacids, aspirins, or non-steroidals should be taken during testing period
- Smoking is not allowed at many centers. If a patient smokes during the study this has to be noted in the diary.

Event buttons
If the ambulatory pressure and pH recorder has event buttons, instruct the patient how to operate these during the study. The buttons are used to mark different periods and events during the study. Examples of event buttons and their functions are given below:

 Chest symptoms such as heartburn/chest pain

 Eating: should mark before and after eating

 Supine: begin and end

 Could mark any other event, such as belching, hiccups, vomiting, coughing, smoking, etc.

Diary

Instruct the patient to also keep a written diary during the study to record meals, sleep, and symptoms, noting their time of occurrence using the time displayed on the equipment

Procedure

1 Calibrate the equipment according to user's manual (both for pH monitoring and pressure monitoring)
2 Put fresh batteries in the recorder
3 Nasally intubate the patient, who should be sitting in an erect position (see Chapter 7): if two catheters are used (one motility and one pH catheter) these can normally be passed, one at a time, through the same nostril
4 Insert the motility or combined motility–pH catheter until the sensors are in the stomach, usually around 60 cm. From this position the catheter is slowly pulled out so that the pressure transducers are placed 3, 8, and 13 cm above the LES. Identification of LES has either been manometrically done prior to the study or may with some equipment be done at this point using an on-line adapter. The actual pressure tracings are then seen on the computer screen while placing the catheter. If a separate pH catheter is used, intubate the catheter through, if possible, the same nostril. Pass the electrode down to the stomach and observe the pH value which verifies the position in the stomach (pH 1–3). Withdraw the pH catheter and position the distal pH sensor 5 cm above the already identified proximal LES border
5 Give the patient 5 ml of room temperature water from a syringe to swallow (wet swallows). Repeat five times at 30-s intervals to verify the motility catheter's position in the esophagus
6 Once the catheter is in the correct position, tape the catheter to the nose. If two catheters are used tape them together. Make a loop of the catheter (catheters) behind the ear. Tape it to the lower part of the neck. Secure with tape in several places
7 If the pH catheter has an external reference attach an adhesive ring on it and apply gel on the gray surface of the reference electrode. Connect the reference on a place where it is less likely to be disturbed by the patient's movements (e.g. the skin of the chest). Make a loop of the cable and secure firmly with tape (Fig. 8.52)
8 Allow the patient to adjust to the catheter (catheters) (5–10 min) before starting the procedure
9 Disconnect the on-line adapter if this has been used. Fasten the probe adapter securely to the recorder
10 Start the recording either at the motility laboratory or instruct the patient how to start the recording when reaching home
11 Send the patient home with written instructions, diary, and an emergency number where the patient can reach the motility nurse or

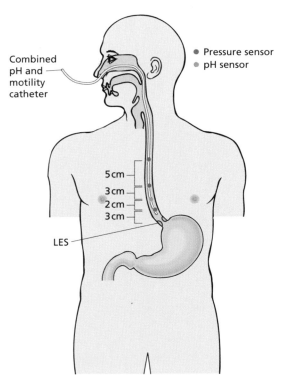

Combined
pH and
motility
catheter

● Pressure sensor
● pH sensor

5 cm
3 cm
2 cm
3 cm

LES

Figure 8.52 Placement of combined pH and motility catheter.

doctor at any time if there are any problems (e.g. if the catheter becomes dislodged)

12 The patient returns to the lab the day after the insertion of the catheter. Recheck the position of the catheter (catheters) and then remove them without turning off the recorder.

An example of a combined esophageal pH and motility study is shown in Fig. 8.53.

After the study
- The patient can resume his/her normal activities and diet and recommence any discontinued medication
- Upload the recorder onto the computer in the lab
- Clean and disinfect the catheter according to hospital regulations and catheter manufacturer's instructions.

chapter 8

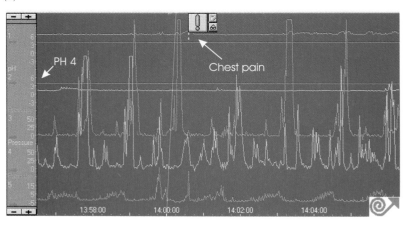

(a)

Esophageal pH

Esophageal pH 5 cm above LES

Esophageal Pressure Ch 3-5

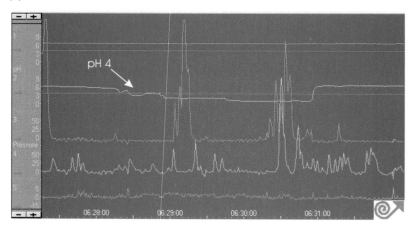

(b)

PH 4

Chest pain

(c)

pH 4

Figure 8.53 Three tracings from a 43-year-old man with a 2 year history of chest pain. (a) Tracing shows the beginning (normal) of an ambulatory 24-h pH and esophageal motility study. Channels 1–2 record esophageal pH (the distal channel (pH) positioned 5 cm above the LES). Three pressure channels with 5 cm spacings are positioned in the esophagus. (b) When the patient indicates chest pain, the recording shows a long duration reflux and disorganized esophageal peristalsis with high amplitude. (c) Prolonged esophageal acid exposure seems to trigger abnormal esophageal peristalsis.

Interpretations

The quantity of data collected during ambulatory 24-h esophageal motility studies are too large to analyze manually. The automated analysis detects four main types of contraction patterns.

Peristaltic contractions. Contractions in two adjacent levels 5 cm apart with a time interval of 0.25–7.0 s.

Simultaneous contractions. Contractions in two adjacent levels 5 cm apart with a time interval of less than 0.25 s.

Isolated contractions. Contractions detected at a single level.

Reversed peristaltic contractions. The direction of the peristaltic wave is reversed (from distal to proximal sensors). The time delay between contractions in two adjacent levels 5 cm apart is between -0.25 and -1.0 s.

All of these contraction types are found in normal controls; however, peristaltic contractions are by far the most common contractions.

Automatic analysis provides a summary table of contraction patterns and the characteristics of the pressure waves (amplitude, duration, area under the wave, and velocity) during supine—including sleeping, meal, post-prandial, and fasting periods.

Symptom correlation. During the study the patient has marked (using the event marker on the equipment) when he/she has felt any symptoms. These symptoms are correlated to abnormal esophageal contraction patterns, and also to esophageal pH < 4. This identifies whether the patient's symptoms are due to esophageal motility disorders or acid gastro-esophageal reflux.

For specific characteristics of esophageal motility disorders, see Section 2.4.

8

chapter

8.6 Advanced UES manometry

UES studies are usually performed as a part of a standard esophageal motility study (see p. 168). However, if oropharyngeal swallowing disorders are suspected, a separate and specific study should be performed. Specific catheters are used and often combined with fluoroscopy.

There are three features of the UES that greatly influence the specific manometric technique:

1 UES moves 2–3 cm orad during a swallow
2 the oval slit-like shape of the UES and its pressure asymmetry
3 the rapidity of the pressure changes in the region of UES which exceed that of any other part of the gastrointestinal tract.

Indications
- Oropharyngeal swallowing disorders
- Zenker's diverticulum.

Contraindications
- See contraindications for nasal intubation (see Chapter 7).

Equipment
- Solid state catheter. The most commonly used type is the Castell-type solid state catheter. The catheter consists of four radioopaque pressure sensors, two distal circumferential sensors which provide a pressure recording over 360°, and two directional sensors measuring 120° (see Fig. 8.54). Compared to a water-perfused catheter it has a faster response time, it does not restrict the patient's position thus allowing the patients to sit erect when swallowing, and perfusion is not involved thus avoiding irritation of the hypopharynx inducing involuntary swallows. Another catheter that may be used in detailed studies of the UES is a solid state catheter with a sleeve sensor (see p. 171)
- Multichannel recording system (Polygraf)
- Personal computer with UES esophageal analysis software
- Printer
- Accessories:

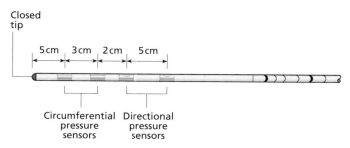

Figure 8.54 Castell-type catheter.

(a) lubricating gel
(b) anesthesia gel
(c) cotton-tip applicators
(d) tape or pHix strips
(e) syringe 10–50 ml
(f) emesis basin
(g) nonsterile gloves
(h) tissues
(i) cup with straw.

Before the study

- 48 h prior to the study the patient should stop taking medications such as:
  (a) nitrates
  (b) calcium channel blockers
  (c) promotility agents
  (d) sedatives
  (e) analgesics
  (f) antidepressants
  (g) H_2-blockers
  (h) antacids (24 h prior to study)
- The patient should fast for at least 6 h prior to the study to decrease the chance of aspiration
- Assess patient information:
  (a) medical history
  (b) symptoms
  (c) medications
  (d) allergies
- Explain the procedure to the patient to increase patient cooperation and comfort level
- Verify signed informed consent (if applicable for the institution).

Procedure

The parameters that should be studied are:
1 UES resting pressure
2 residual pressure during UES relaxation both for wet and dry swallows
3 duration of UES relaxation
4 UES contraction pressure
5 pharyngeal pressure at the level of the inferior pharyngeal constrictor
6 pharyngeal pressure at the location of the tongue base.

UES RESTING PRESSURE

1 The catheter is nasally intubated with the patient sitting erect (see Chapter 7). All pressure channels should be positioned in the esophagus
2 The patient should be sitting during the entire UES study

189

3 Identify the HPZ of the UES by performing a slow pull through of the UES

4 Starting in the most distal part, withdraw the catheter in 0.5–1 cm steps waiting 10 s without catheter manipulation or swallowing at each station. Be aware that the proximal transducers are positioned with the recording sites in a dorsal direction. (The catheter assembly incorporates a marker outside the nares which indicates sensor orientation)

5 The highest UES pressure found (mid- or end-respiratory pressure) is referred to as the UES resting pressure

6 UES resting pressure should be registered at the beginning of the study, and also at the end of the examination when the patient is more relaxed.

RESIDUAL PRESSURE DURING UES RELAXATION BOTH FOR WET AND DRY SWALLOWS

1 Position the catheter sensor in (or slightly above) the proximal part of the UES to avoid UES moving above the sensor on laryngeal elevation when swallowing. If the latter occurs esophageal pressure will be measured instead of UES pressure

2 The catheter may either be fluoroscopically or manometrically positioned (slow pull through as above)

3 Give the patient a bolus of 5 ml room temperature water from a syringe to achieve wet swallows. Mark each wet swallow directly on the computer screen

4 Do a series of 10 wet swallows waiting at least 20–30 s between swallows

5 If required, do a series of *dry* swallows waiting at least 20–30 s between swallows. Mark the tracing at each dry swallow

When swallowing, the recording shows an M-shaped configuration (Fig 8.55) due to:

• an increase in pressure as the HPZ moves orad onto the transducer

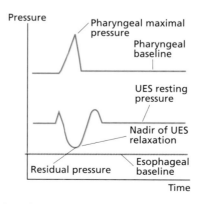

Figure 8.55 The M-shaped UES relaxation.

- a fall in pressure as the UES relaxes
- an increase in pressure as the UES closes
- a decrease in pressure as the UES returns to its initial position.

DURATION OF UES RELAXATION

The duration of UES relaxation can easily be calculated when analyzing the recording of the UES relaxation.

UES CONTRACTION PRESSURE

This is the contraction pressure in the UES when the peristaltic wave reaches the UES. UES contraction is an integrated part of pharyngeal peristalsis and contributes to bolus transport through the UES.

PHARYNGEAL PRESSURE AT THE INFERIOR PHARYNGEAL CONSTRICTOR

1 When the distal circumferential sensor is positioned at or slightly above the orad border of the UES, the sensor 3 cm orad to the distal circumferential sensor will pick up the pharyngeal contraction at the level of the inferior pharyngeal constrictor
2 If the pressure level in the recording reaches values as high as 600 mmHg or so, this is almost certainly an artifact. The pressure is then created when the epiglottis tilts down and hits the sensor. Small adjustments of the sensor position can overcome the artifact.

PHARYNGEAL PRESSURE AT THE BASE OF THE TONGUE

With the catheter in the same position as above, the sensor 5 cm orad to the distal circumferential sensor will pick up the pharyngeal contraction pressures at this level.

COORDINATION OF PERISTALTIC CONTRACTIONS IN THE PHARYNX AND RELAXATION OF THE UES

1 The coordination of pharyngeal contraction and UES relaxation may be studied by analyzing the wet and dry swallow procedure (see above)
2 Coordination is one of the most important features to study in patients with dysphagia. Normally pharynx contraction should occur simultaneously with the nadir of relaxation.

INTRABOLUS PRESSURE AT INFERIOR PHARYNGEAL CONSTRICTOR

Elevated intrabolus pressure has been postulated as an important factor in UES dysfunction.

Pharyngeal manometry can be performed during a barium swallow (e.g. synchronized digital imaging). The pressure registered when the manometric sensor is surrounded by fluid (the intrabolus pressure) is measured.

If intrabolus pressure is elevated despite complete UES relaxation, this verifies a decreased compliance of the UES. Complete manometric relaxation of the UES is not followed by complete opening of the sphincter. The elevated intrabolus pressure compensates for the lack of compliance.

After the study
- Remove the catheter from the patient
- Obtain and document the patient's vital signs
- Instruct the patient that a cold gargle may be used for minor throat irritation
- The patient can resume his/her normal activities and restart any discontinued medications
- Clean and disinfect the catheter according to hospital regulations and catheter manufacturer's instructions.

Interpretations
Incomplete relaxation of UES is a feature of many neurologic diseases including cerebrovascular accidents, Parkinson's disease, poliomyelitis, trauma (head injuries, iatrogenic nerve injuries).

Pharyngeal weakness may be a result of neurologic or muscle diseases, surgical scarring or radiation therapy.

Reduced compliance of UES has been demonstrated in patients with Zenker's diverticulum.

Dyscoordination of pharyngeal contractions and UES relaxation is a common cause of dysphagia. The lack of coordination can be due to many different neurologic and muscle diseases.

Examples of tracings. See Figs 8.56–8.58.

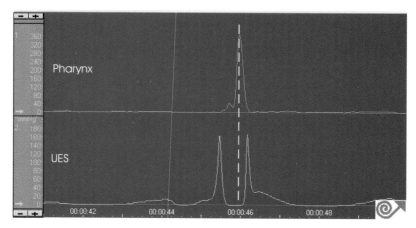

Figure 8.56 Normal UES manometry. The cursor shows normal coordination between the pharyngeal spike and the UES relaxation.

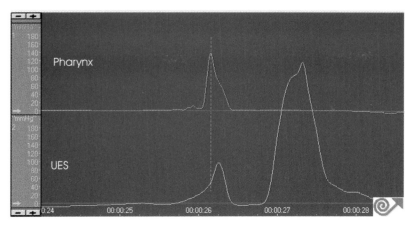

Figure 8.57 Tracing from a patient with Parkinson's disease who has swallowing difficulties. UES manometry shows poor coordination between the pharyngeal spike and the UES relaxation.

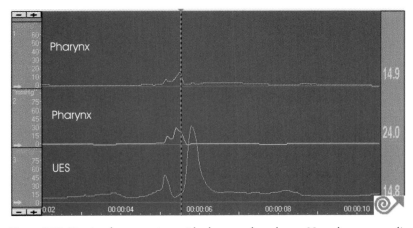

Figure 8.58 Tracing from a patient with pharyngeal weakness. Note the poor amplitude of the pharyngeal contractions but normal coordination between pharyngeal spikes and UES relaxation.

Pitfalls

- UES resting pressure is markedly asymmetric with greater values anteriorly and posteriorly compared to values measured laterally. This asymmetry is due to the slit-like configuration of the sphincter. Be aware of the direction of the sensors. This problem is avoided by using a sleeve catheter which assembly positions itself in the correct anterioposterior position
- The technique of measurement itself stimulates sphincter contraction. The less movement applied to the catheter, the lower the recorded pressures
- In patients with Zenker's diverticulum be aware that the manometric catheter may curl in the pharyngeal pouch instead of progressing down the esophagus.

193

8.7 Antroduodenal manometry

Indications

This procedure is still mainly used as a research tool; however, there are some clinical indications:

- to diagnose or exclude chronic intestinal pseudoobstruction (CIP)
- in patients with systemic diseases that may affect gastrointestinal motility (e.g. diabetes mellitus, progressive systemic sclerosis) to define intestinal involvement
- postviral gastroparesis and dysmotility syndromes
- preoperative evaluation of CIP patients being considered for intestinal transplantation
- in the assessment of patients with severe idiopathic dyspeptic symptoms such as pain, nausea, and vomiting—but without evidence of organic diseases
- predictions of drug effect—the acute effect of prokinetic drugs (e.g. cisapride, metoclopramide, domperidone, and erythromycin) can be ascertained during motility tests
- to determine optimal approach for enteric feeding (oral, gastric, or jejunal).

Contraindications

- See contraindications for nasal intubation (see Chapter 7).

Equipment

- Catheter: solid state or perfused multilumen catheter. The advantages of using a solid state catheter compared to a water-perfused catheter are that the placement of the catheter beyond the pylorus into the duodenum is often easier since it is stiffer, and that the patient does not need to be completely still during the study
- The configuration of the catheter may vary considerably depending on individual requirements, but it often includes at least three channels which is sufficient to determine migrating motor complex (MMC). Distances between recording sites must be based on the purpose of the test. In antroduodenal coordination studies and distal antral contraction studies channels need to be, at most, 1 cm apart
- Multiple channel recording system (e.g. Polygraf in stationary motility studies) or ambulatory data recorder
- If a perfused catheter is to be used, a hydraulic capillary infusion system is needed. Infusion rate depends on the catheter lumen (common infusion rate in adult antroduodenal manometry is 0.25 ml/min). External pressure transducer for each channel
- Personal computer
- Analysis software

- Accessories:
  - (a) lubricating gel
  - (b) anesthetic gel
  - (c) cotton-tip applicators
  - (d) emesis basin
  - (e) nonsterile gloves
  - (f) tissues
  - (g) cup with straw.

Before the study

- Assess patient information:
  - (a) medical history
  - (b) symptoms
  - (c) medications
  - (d) allergies
- Verify signed informed consent (if applicable for the institution)
- All medications that could interfere with the motility study should stop 48 h prior to the study (calcium blockers, adrenergic agents, tricyclic antidepressants, opioids)
- Study should be performed after an overnight fast in order to avoid aspiration due to intubation and to be certain that fasting motor patterns (the MMC) may be recorded
- If the patient is on parenteral nutrition stop nutrients and replace with crystalloids 12 h prior to starting the procedure
- Explain the procedure to the patient to obtain patient cooperation and increase comfort level
- Sedation should not routinely be given. If needed, sedation with IV midazolam (2–5 mg) followed by reversal with flumazenil (0.2–0.4 mg) can be used. Wait 1 h before starting the study to allow for drug metabolism.

Procedure

1 Intubate the patient through the nose (see Chapter 7). Have the patient lie in a right lateral position with bended knees in order to facilitate passage of catheter beyond the pylorus into the duodenum. Solid state catheters are usually stiff enough to be easily guided beyond the pylorus into the duodenum. A guidewire may be used when placing softer perfused catheters in the duodenum. A steerable catheter or upper gastrointestinal endoscopy may be used to place the guidewire with its tip beyond the angle of Treitz

2 Fluoroscopy is an accurate method to aid and verify catheter placement. It ensures that the sensors are at the desired location; which may be difficult especially when placing sensors across the antroduodenal junction. If normal placement of catheter fails, endoscopic catheter placement may be used for exact positioning. In this case as little air as possible must be delivered since distention of the intestinal wall affects motility. By

8

chapter

checking the motility pattern the duodenal placement of the catheter can be confirmed. In antroduodenal manometry studies, one or two recording sites are often positioned in the antrum and the remainder in the duodenum. The most distal sensor is then normally positioned at the ligament of Treitz. In small bowel studies the middle sensor is normally positioned at the ligament of Treitz

3 Position of patient: in stationary studies with perfused catheters, let the patient lie comfortably. Provide magazines and books to occupy the patient. In ambulatory recordings, solid state catheters are used, and the patient is free to move around as he/she wishes and may also leave the hospital and return in time for removal of the catheter

4 For ambulatory settings have the patient keep a diary during the study to record meals, sleep, position, and symptoms, noting their time of occurrence using the time displayed on the ambulatory recorder. Ambulatory recordings have the advantage of providing information on daytime fasting and fed motility, and also nocturnal fasting motility

5 Recordings should be performed for at least 6 h in stationary studies to determine the presence of MMC—phase 3. Ambulatory recordings up to 24 h

6 Provocation with infusion of erythromycin or SC injection of octreotide may be used. Intravenous erythromycin induces a phase 3-like complex in healthy subjects

7 Postprandial motility should also be evaluated. A meal inhibits the MMC and induces a postprandial motility pattern. A test meal can be given once the MMC has been determined

8 The stationary study is usually performed 4 h fasting and then 2 h postprandially.

After the study

- Remove the catheter from the patient
- Obtain and document the patient's vital signs
- Instruct the patient that a cold gargle may be used for minor throat irritation
- The patient can resume his/her normal activities and restart any discontinued medications
- Clean and disinfect the catheter according to hospital regulations and catheter manufacturer's instructions.

Interpretations

Normal antroduodenal manometry is shown in Fig. 8.59.

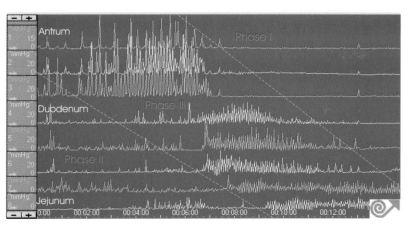

Figure 8.59 Normal antroduodenal manometry showing MMC with its different phases.

NEUROPATHIC PROCESSES

A variety of diseases affecting the enteric, autonomic or central nervous system such as visceral CIP, multiple sclerosis, diabetes mellitus, Parkinson's disease, disorders of the brainstem, and viruses (e.g. herpes, varicella zoster, Epstein–Barr) may cause antroduodenal motility abnormalities (Fig. 8.60) such as:

- increased frequency of fasting MMCs while awake
- disrupted MMC activity
- postprandial hypomotility
- a rapid return to MMC activity (within 2 h) after a meal of more than 500 kcal.

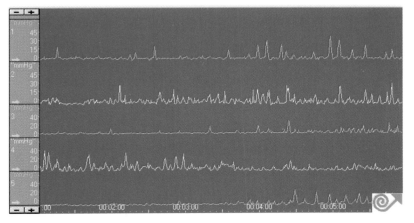

Figure 8.60 Antroduodenal manometry in patient with neuropathic pseudoobstruction showing a disorganized poor propagating phase III pattern and rapid propagation of abnormal contractions.

MYOPATHIC DISORDERS

A variety of myopathic disorders such as myogenic pseudoobstruction, amyloidosis, collagen vascular diseases, and muscular dystrophies may cause motility abnormalities (Fig. 8.61) including low-amplitude contractile (including MMC) activity at the affected sites. (Ensure that obstruction has been excluded since low-amplitude MMCs are seen proximal to the site of obstruction, see Fig. 8.62).

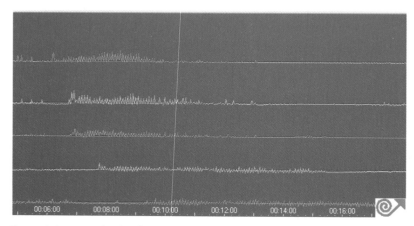

Figure 8.61 Antroduodenal manometry in patient with myopathic pseudoobstruction showing an MMC of low amplitude.

GASTROPARESIS

There is antral hypomotility shown by:
- reduced postprandial frequency of distal antral contractions or
- reduced postprandial frequency of common cavity antral contractions extending over 6 cm from the pylorus.

MECHANICAL OBSTRUCTION OF THE SMALL INTESTINE

This occurrence should, of course, be diagnosed by radiologic means. However, manometry will show a specific pattern (Fig. 8.62):
- simultaneous prolonged contractions
- clustered minute contractions separated by periods of quiescence (significant if observed postprandially for over 30 min).

CHRONIC DYSPEPSIA PATIENTS

- Postprandial hypomotility in the antrum—the frequency and amplitude of the contractions is less in patients with dyspepsia compared to healthy people. This can lead to delayed gastric emptying which is also common in patients with functional dyspepsia
- Phase 3 of the MMC in the stomach is often missing in dyspepsia patients
- Duodenal motility disturbances are also common (Fig. 8.63).

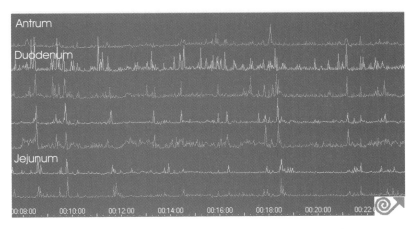

Figure 8.62 Antroduodenal manometry showing discrete clusters of contractions resulting from mechanical obstruction of a healthy gut.

PEPTIC ULCER DISEASE

- Reduction of MMC activity in a gastric ulcer which persists after healing suggests an impaired antropyloric motor function (primary or secondary)
- Antropyloroduodenal motor function disruption has also been described in duodenal ulcers but its significance is unclear.

POSTTRUNCAL VAGOTOMY

- Impaired fed pattern
- Suppression of antral MMC

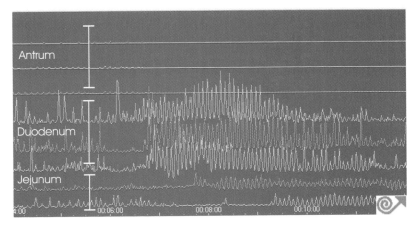

Figure 8.63 Antroduodenal manometry in a patient with dyspepsia. In dyspepsia patients the phase 3 activity of the MMC is more often absent in the antral channels than in normals.

- Receptive relaxation in the fundus is abolished. This results in increased gastric tone which increases the rate of initial emptying. This may cause dumping
- Ectopic pacemakers develop in the distal stomach and fire at rates of 4/min or greater, override the normal rhythm and cause tachygastria.

MOTILITY ABNORMALITIES

The following is a list of antroduodenal motility abnormalities and the diseases/disorders in which they may occur.

Phase 3 absent or less frequent

- Idiopathic delayed gastric emptying
- Orthostatic hypotension
- Systemic sclerosis
- Diabetic gastroparesis
- Pseudoobstruction
- Duodenal and gastric ulcer disease.

Short interval between phase 3

- CIP
- Irritable bowel syndrome with diarrhea
- Short bowel syndrome
- Diabetic motility disorders
- Postvagotomy diarrhea.

Abnormal propagation of phase 3 (nonpropagating, retrograde, and slowly propagating phase 3)

- Functional upper gut symptoms
- Myotonic dystrophy
- CIP
- Brainstem encephalitis
- Bacterial overgrowth.

Frequent nonmigrating clusters of contraction

- Pseudoobstruction
- Orthostatic hypotension
- Diabetic gastroparesis
- Mechanical obstruction
- Systemic sclerosis
- Functional upper gut symptoms
- Some cases of chronic diarrhea.

Failure to change to postprandial activity

- Pseudoobstruction
- Diabetic gastroparesis

Postprandial duodenal hypomotility
- Pseudoobstruction
- Antral hypomotility
- Functional upper gut symptoms
- Systemic sclerosis
- Orthostatic hypotension
- Diabetic gastroparesis
- Myotonic dystrophy (in adults).

Pitfalls

- Several dysmotility syndromes may share common pathophysiology (see diseases listed above). There are interpretive limitations due to the limited motor repertoire in the gut
- The link between specific pathology, symptoms, and motor abnormality has not yet been fully demonstrated
- Stress may cause abnormal motor patterns (delayed gastric emptying, impaired antral contractility, suppression of MMC cycling, induction of irregular patterns)
- The possible effects of intravenous infusions must be taken into account. High blood glucose levels (higher than 140 mg/dl) reduce the occurrence of gastric phase 3. Also hyperglycemia inhibits gastric emptying.

An algorithm of the clinical syndromes suggestive of a motility disorder is given in Fig. 8.64.

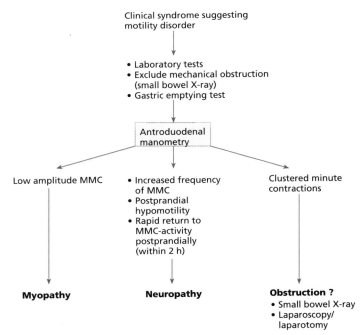

Figure 8.64 Algorithm showing the investigation of a clinical syndrome suggestive of a motility disorder.

8.8 Electrogastrography

Electrogastrography (EGG) detects abnormal gastric myoelectrical rhythms. This equipment has mainly been used in research so far, but there are indications that this may be a useful clinical tool in the future.

Indications

- Gastroparesis
- Evaluation of patients with symptoms suggestive of gastric dysmotility (nausea, vomiting, postprandial abdominal pain, postprandial abdominal bloating/distention)
- To monitor the effects of medications (antiemetic or prokinetic therapy) on gastric myoelectric activity
- In patients with symptoms related to other parts of the gastrointestinal tract to determine if there is also a gastric motor function abnormality:
  (a) in patients with chronic constipation to detect if there is any extra-colonic involvement
  (b) in patients with GERD to assess if gastroparesis is a contributing factor to GERD
  (c) to predict those who may have problems after Nissen fundoplication
  (d) to assess those with vomiting and nausea after fundoplication.

Contraindications

If the patient is not capable of sitting or lying still.

Equipment (Fig. 8.65)

- EGG recorder
- Skin abrasive gel
- Adhesive gel EGG electrodes

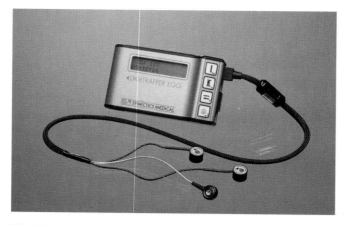

Figure 8.65 EGG equipment.

- Skin conductive cream
- IBM-compatible personal computer
- Software analysis program
- Several gauze 4 × 4 pads
- Simple battery powered Ohm-meter (optional).

Before the study

- Study performed in the morning after an overnight fast
- All drugs known to alter gastric myoelectric activity are discontinued 48 h prior to the study
- Explain the procedure to the patient to increase patient cooperation and comfort level
- Verify signed informed consent (if applicable for the institution)
- Instruct the patient to pay attention to potential electrical or radio interferences (neon, cellular phones, etc.).

During the study

- The patient should be in a reclined comfortable position to help eliminate motion artifacts
- Patient must not talk or move during study
- Patient can read quietly or watch TV.

Procedure

1 Shave abdominal hair at sites for electrodes
2 Prepare the skin by abrasion with abrasive gel (Omni-Prep)
3 Administer electrode conductive cream. Rub it in, and let it dry for 1 min
4 Rub away any excess conductive cream from electrode area with a dry gauze
5 Place the EGG electrodes close to the antral region along the antral axis of the stomach. One electrode on the patient's ventral mid-line, halfway between the xyphoid process and umbilicus. The other active electrode on the patient's left side, 5 cm distant and 45° superiorly. The electrode for the reference lead is positioned on the patient's right side, 10–15 cm distant and at the same level/plane as the middle electrode (Fig. 8.66)
6 Use Ohm-meter to test electrode impedance. If less than 5 kOhm, proceed with EGG study. If greater than 5 kOhm and skin in the electrode areas is not pink from abrasion, repeat the skin preparation procedure using new EGG electrodes
7 Record while fasting for 30–60 min
8 Give the patient a standardized test meal (e.g. egg sandwich with 200 ml water). Mark beginning and end of meal. On some equipment there is an event button to press
9 Record the postprandial signal for another 60–90 min
10 Terminate the recording, and disconnect the patient from the electrodes.

8

chapter

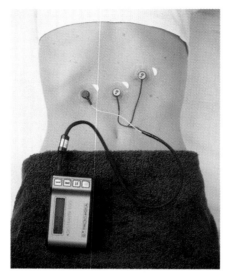

Figure 8.66 Position of EGG electrodes.

After the study

- Remove the electrodes, and wipe the abdomen
- Patient may resume his/her normal activities and restart any discontinued medication
- Upload the recording into the computer.

Interpretations

- Normally, there is an increase in signal power or amplitude after meal ingestion
- The ratio of the postprandial power of the dominant frequency to the pre-prandial power of the dominant frequency can be calculated. Normally, the postprandial to fasting power ratio is greater than 1. A ratio less than 1 is abnormal and suggests decreased motor response to a meal, and/or distention of the stomach in fasting state and with no further gastric distention on meal ingestion
- The dominant frequency is normally between 2 and 4 cycles/min for at least 75% of the postprandial period
- Both tachygastria (over 4 cycles/min) and bradygastria (less than 2 cycles/min) have been associated with antral hypomotility
- All the patterns of gastric dysrhythmia (bradygastria, tachygastria, mixed patterns, or flat pattern—absent activity) have been observed in patients with:
  (a) idiopathic gastroparesis
  (b) diabetic gastroparesis
  (c) nausea of pregnancy
  (d) motion sickness
  (e) unexplained nausea and vomiting—dyspepsia (in absence of altered gastric emptying)

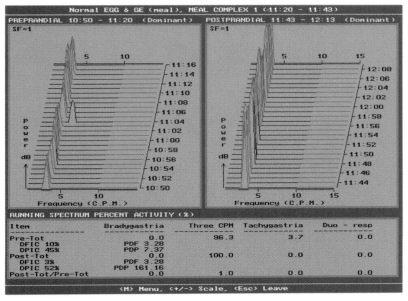

(a)

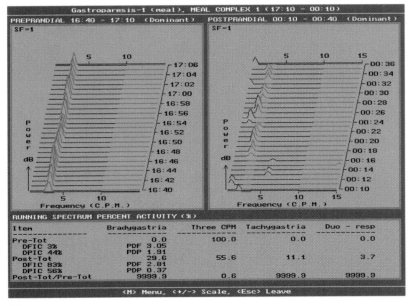

(b)

Figure 8.67 Examples of EGG with fast Fourier analysis in a healthy individual (a) and in a patient with gastroparesis (b). In the healthy individual there is an increase in signal power/amplitude postprandially; the dominant frequency is 3 cpm. In the patient with gastroparesis there is no increase in signal power/amplitude in response to a solid meal; the dominant frequency postprandially is abnormal with both tachy- and bradygastria.

205

Table 8.4 Many disorders produce gastric dysrhythmia such as tachygastria and/or bradygastria or a mixture of both (tachyarrhythmia).

Diseases	Bradygastria 1–2 cycles/min	Tachygastria 4–9 cycles/min	Tachyarrhythmia
Gastroparesis	+	+	+
Chronic intestinal pseudoobstruction	+	+	
Functional dyspepsia: dysmotility type with normal gastric emptying	+	+	+
Bulimia nervosa	+		
Anorexia nervosa		+	
Drug-induced (e.g. epinephrine, morphine sulfate)	+	+	
Postoperative ileus, cholecystectomy, Roux-en-Y	+		
Premature infants		+	
Motion sickness			+
Nausea of pregnancy	+	+	+

- Gastroparesis is associated with EGG abnormalities (Fig. 8.67) such as:
  (a) abnormal dominant frequency in either the fasting or the fed state. High percentage of time in bradygastria and/or tachygastria (Table 8.4)
  (b) decreased postprandial to preprandial power ratio after a solid meal.

Pitfalls

- If recording time is too short, transient dysrhythmia may not occur
- Motion artifacts may look like dysrhythmic activity (Fig. 8.68)
- Registration of colonic signals
- Superimposition of duodenal rhythm (10–12 cpm)
- Poor skin preparation will greatly exaggerate any artifacts from patient motion or ambient electrical interference (e.g. cellular phones).

Algorithm for diagnosis is shown in Fig. 8.69.

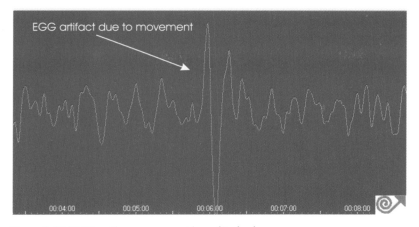

Figure 8.68 EGG artifact seen as rapid amplitude change.

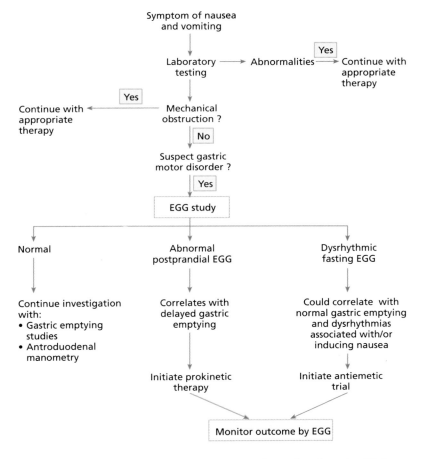

Figure 8.69 Suggested algorithm for the diagnosis of a GI disorder using EGG as a clinical tool.

207

8.9 Ambulatory gamma counting

The assessment of gastric motility is important in the evaluation of patients with foregut symptoms. One important diagnostic endpoint is the measurement of gastric emptying.

In clinical practice gastric emptying is assessed by the scintigraphic measurement of the emptying of a radiolabeled test meal in a standard position using gamma camera scanning. Repetitive measurements of gastric emptying in the same patient under different physiologic conditions are more sensitive in detecting abnormal gastric emptying patterns than a single measurement in a standard position.

Recently an ambulatory gamma counting probe has been successfully used for the measurement of gastric emptying in normal volunteers and patients with foregut symptoms. This probe has been shown to facilitate repetitive measurements under different physiologic conditions in the same individual by using ambulatory equipment.

This equipment has so far mainly been used in research, but there are indications that it may be a useful clinical tool in the future.

Indications
- Gastric symptoms following previous foregut surgery
- GERD and gastric symptoms
- Diabetes mellitus and gastric symptoms
- Nonulcer dyspepsia (gastric symptoms in the presence of no mucosal lesion on upper endoscopy and no functional abnormality on other functional foregut tests)
- Monitoring the effectiveness of prokinetic therapy
- Whenever gastroparesis is suspected.

Equipment
- LES identifier or equipment for stationary esophageal manometry
- Cadmium telluride gamma counting probe
- Preamplifier
- Ambulatory data recorder (e.g. Synectics ambulatory gamma counter (Fig. 8.70))
- Computer, software, printer
- Material for transnasal intubation
- Access to a standardized radiolabeled test meal (one scrambled egg labeled with 1 mCi ^{99m}Tc with two slices of white bread and 100 ml of tap water).

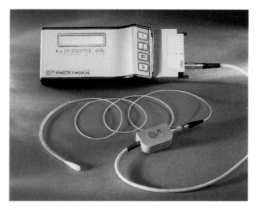

Figure 8.70 The Synectics ambulatory gamma counter.

Before the study

- Discontinue all medication known to interfere with gastric motor function at least 3 days before the study or depending on the washout of the medication
- No food intake at least 8 h before the start of the study
- Determine the lower border of the LES with the LES identifier in the ambulatory recorder or by stationary esophageal manometry
- Mark the probe cable at a position bringing the tip of the probe 5 cm below the lower border of the LES
- Set up the recorder for the gastric emptying study.

Proposed study protocol

- *7:30 a.m.* Intubation with the cadmium-telluride gamma detecting probe and positioning of the tip of the probe 5 cm below the lower border of the LES (for details see Section 8.1). Once the probe is inserted:
  (a) secure the probe cable to the patient's nose at the position of the marker
  (b) connect the probe cable to the preamplifier
  (c) attach the preamplifier to a rope around the patient's shoulder
  (d) connect the preamplifier to the data recorder
- *8:00 a.m.* The first of three identical test meals is given. The patient stays sitting for 3 h following test meal ingestion
- *12:00 noon* The second of three identical test meals is given. The patient is positioned on a stretcher in a semireclining position (30° head up position) for 3 h following test meal ingestion
- *4:00 p.m.* The third of three identical test meals is given. The patient is either standing or walking for 2.5 h following test meal ingestion
- *6:30 p.m.* The probe is removed and the test is complete.

209

During the study

- Before each of the three identical test meals is ingested the patient should be allowed to use the bathroom, so that the same measurement position can be maintained over the complete 3-h measurement period following each meal
- The patient should have at least 30 min break in between meals
- All test meals should be chewed well and ingested within 5 min
- No additional foods or drinks are allowed during the study.

After the study

- Clean the gamma detector probe with water and disinfect the probe according to hospital regulations and catheter manufacturer's instructions directly after the study
- Download the recorded data into the gastric emptying analysis software according to the software manual instructions
- The patient can resume his/her normal activities and diet and restart any discontinued medication.

Interpretation

The data obtained with the intraluminal probe are downloaded on a personal computer and evaluated using the software for ambulatory gamma counting. The data are corrected to take account of decay of the isotope. The area under the decay corrected data curve is calculated for 18 consecutive 10-min intervals starting at the end of the test meal ingestion T_0 (Fig. 8.71).

The interval with the maximum activity is defined as 100%, and the activity in the remaining intervals is expressed as a percentage of this maximum activity. This results in 18 consecutive values for the percentage radioactivity retained with the stomach. The emptying half-time can be extrapolated from this curve.

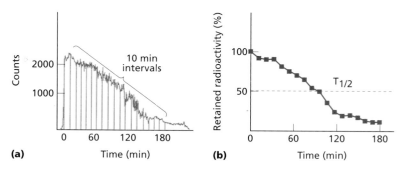

Figure 8.71 Graphs showing (a) decay of ingested isotope with time after ingestion of meal, (b) percentage radioactivity retained within the stomach at times after ingestion.

The radioactivity retained within the stomach at each consecutive 10-min interval is compared to the 5th and 95th percentiles for the radioactivity retained within the stomach at the corresponding 10-min intervals in 30 normal volunteers.

Delayed gastric emptying
When the radioactivity retained within the stomach exceeds the 95th percentile of these normal volunteers during three or more consecutive 10-min intervals starting 90 min after the onset of measurement.

Rapid gastric emptying
When the radioactivity retained within the stomach is less than the 5th percentile of normal volunteers during two or more consecutive 10-min intervals within the first 60 min of measurement.

The normal ranges for the three different measurement positions (Fig. 8.72) according to the protocol outlined above are included in the ambulatory gamma counting software.

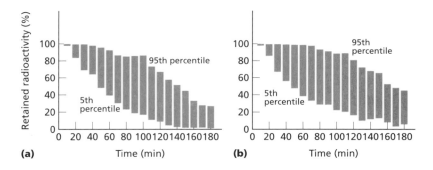

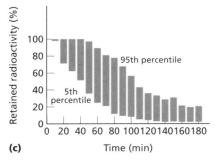

Figure 8.72 Normal ranges of retained radioactivity with time in (a) sitting measurement position, (b) semireclining measurement position, and (c) standing/walking measurement position.

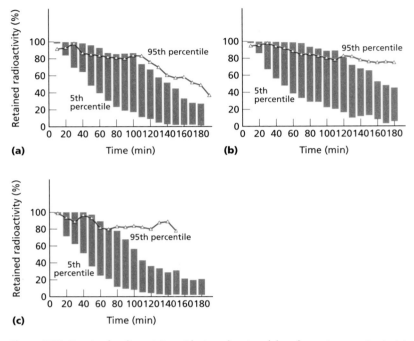

Figure 8.73 Retained radioactivity with time showing delayed gastric emptying in (a) sitting position, (b) semireclining position, and (c) standing/walking position in a patient with previous Bilroth I gastrectomy.

The three repetitive measurements under three different physiologic conditions allow a grading of gastric dysfunction in that patients with the most severe dysfunction usually demonstrate abnormal gastric emptying patterns following two or all three test meals, while patients with a mild gastric motility disorder may have delayed or rapid gastric emptying following one meal and normal gastric emptying patterns following the other two meals. Based on this the patient's therapy can be adjusted to the degree of gastric dysmotility. Figure 8.73 shows the tracings obtained from a patient after previous Billroth I partial gastrectomy with severe gastric stasis and delayed gastric emptying in all three meals.

Figure 8.74 was obtained in a patient with multiple previous gastric surgeries and postprandial dumping symptoms. Rapid gastric emptying patterns are observed following the meal in the sitting and standing/walking postures while the emptying following the meal in the semireclining position was still within the normal range.

chapter

8

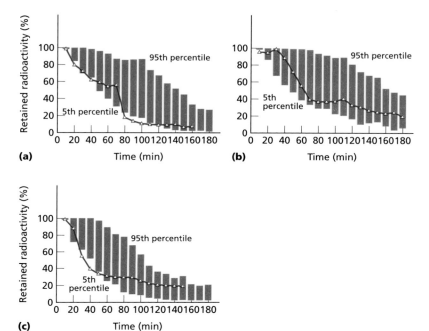

Figure 8.74 Retained radioactivity with time in a patient with multiple gastric surgeries and postprandial dumping syndrome in (a) sitting position showing borderline rapid gastric emptying, (b) semireclining position showing normal gastric emptying and (c) standing/walking position showing rapid gastric emptying.

8

chapter

8.10 Anorectal manometry

Indications

- Constipation
- Fecal incontinence
- For evaluation prior to medical intervention, surgery, or biofeedback
- Pre- and postoperative evaluation.

Equipment

- Either (i) anorectal small balloon motility probe (one perfused lumen located 1 cm from distal tip for measuring rectal pressures and three latex balloons, one for distending the rectum and two for measuring pressures in the anal canal); or (ii) standard perfusion catheter with four to eight recording sites radially arranged at 45–90° intervals 7 cm from the tip and one balloon for distending the rectum; or (iii) solid state anorectal catheter with four pressure channels and one balloon for rectal distention studies; and/or (iv) vector volume catheter—six to eight recording sites radially arranged at 45/60° intervals 5 cm from the tip (Fig. 8.75)
- Multichannel recording system (Polygraf)
- Perfusion pump, external pressure transducers (not needed if solid state catheter is used)
- IBM-compatible personal computer
- Software—anorectal manometry analysis

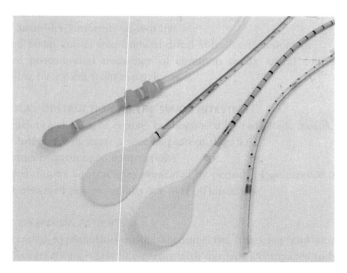

Figure 8.75 Different types of anorectal motility catheters. *From left to right:* small balloon motility probe from Marquat; water-perfused anorectal motility catheter from Zinetics; solid-state 4D anorectal motility catheter; water-perfused vector volume catheter from Zinetics.

- Together with the Polygraf the visceral stimulator/barostat may also be used, with its specific catheter, for anorectal manometry
- Defecation dynamics may be studied by synchronizing manometry, EMG, and videodefecography
- Accessories:
  (a) lubricating gel
  (b) 4 × 4 gauzes
  (c) gloves
  (d) 60 or 100 ml syringe
  (e) towels and washcloth
  (f) three-way stopcocks
  (g) blue pads.

Before the study

- Obtain patient data: symptoms (constipation, urinary or fecal incontinence, perineal or abdominal pain), allergies, past treatments (anal surgery), pelvic trauma
- Written consent is signed if the institution requires it
- No special preparation of the bowel unless the patient has severe constipation with an impaction. Enema may be necessary in this case
- The patient should void residual urine and feces completely before the study
- No sedation is given to the patient
- Explain the procedure to the patient in order to increase patient cooperation and comfort level
- Calibrate equipment according to user's manual.

Procedure

Six important parameters are studied during anorectal manometry:

- maximal voluntary squeeze pressure—external anal sphincter and puborectalis muscle function
- push/strain pressures
- rest/relax pressures
- internal anal sphincter inhibitory reflex to rectal distention (RAIR)
- The rectal volume sensory thresholds. The threshold of first sensation—the ability to sense small volumes of rectal distention, to the threshold of maximum tolerable distention
- Defecation dynamics

Optional parameters are:

- sphincter length
- vector volume analysis of the anal canal.

The procedure is as follows:

1 Patient should be positioned on their left side, with hips and knees flexed. Place a blue pad under the left hip

8

chapter

215

2 Insert well-lubricated manometric catheter into the rectum. Placement depends on the type of probe used (Fig. 8.76). If an anorectal small balloon probe is used, the proximal annular balloon (external anal sphincter balloon) should barely disappear into the anal canal. If a perfusion probe or a solid state catheter is used, the probe should be inserted to a depth of 6 cm from the anal verge

3 Allow the patient to adjust to the catheter before starting the procedure. Wait at least 2–10 min

4 Obtain a recording with a stable baseline in the rectum and/or the anal canal. This is important since all of subsequent measurements will be referred to it. Note if there are any ultra slow waves and spontaneous contractions or relaxations. If the patient moves or talks, etc., note it on the tracing as an artifact. The resting pressure of the anal sphincter can be measured at the start of the procedure or later in the procedure when the patient is thought to be more relaxed.

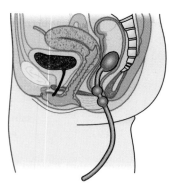

Figure 8.76 Placement of anorectal small balloon catheter.

PROCEDURE WITH ANORECTAL SMALL BALLOON PROBE

1 **The maximal voluntary squeeze pressure**

Have the patient squeeze as hard as possible (as if to hold back stool) for 10–20 s. The external anal sphincter should normally stay contracted for at least 3–5 s. Less than 3 s is considered abnormal. Repeat the squeeze procedure once or twice with more than 30 s between squeezes. Note any artifacts that may occur because the patient moved his/her legs, tilted his/her pelvis, or contracted the buttocks during the squeeze.

2 **The push/strain maneuver**

Ask the patient to push/strain as if trying to defecate. Repeat once or twice with more than 30 s between pushes. The external anal sphincter should normally relax during this maneuver. However, many laboratories have found it difficult for patients to perform this test correctly due to embarrassment in the testing environment. This test is therefore considered optional.

3 Rest/relax maneuver

Let the patient rest quietly with no squeeze or straining for 20–30 s to obtain the resting pressures.

4 Cough maneuver

Is performed in some centers to see if the external anal sphincter contracts in response to a sudden increase in abdominal pressure. Ask the patient to cough. Repeat once or twice with more than 20 s between coughs.

5 Rectoanal inhibitory reflex

This is also called the rectosphincteric reflex and is elicited by distention of the rectum. The minimal volume required to elicit the internal anal sphincter relaxation is defined.

Inflate the rectal balloon with 10 ml of air or body temperature water. Within 3–5 s of inflation the air or water should be completely withdrawn.

Repeat the inflation and increase the volume by 10 ml each time until the RAIR is obtained. Normally a testing sequence of 10, 20, 30, 40, and 50 ml is enough to elicit the RAIR. However, in patients with megarectum much larger volumes may be needed.

After each distention the inflated volume should be documented, regardless of whether or not the patient sensed the balloon, or the RAIR was present or absent.

The internal anal sphincter should normally relax (decrease in pressure 10–15 mmHg) in response to a 50-ml balloon distention.

6 Rectal volume sensory thresholds

The first volume of rectal distention that the patient can distinguish to the maximum tolerable volume is determined.

Inflate 10 ml of water at body temperature into the rectal balloon over 5 s. Wait 20 s and ask the patient what he/she felt. Did he/she feel anything, and was the sensation temporary or constant?

Fill the rectal balloon in increments, allowing a 20 s accommodation period between inflations.

Patient's response to distention is noted by marking each distention: 0 = no sensation, 1 = first sensation, 2 = constant sensation/urge, 3 = maximum tolerable sensation.

PROCEDURE WITH RADIAL PERFUSED OR SOLID STATE CATHETER

1 If a regular radial water-perfused probe or solid state probe is used, instead of a small balloon probe, the first three maneuvers mentioned above (i.e. squeeze, push/strain, and rest/relax maneuvers) should be repeated for every centimeter as the probe is withdrawn in 1 cm increments. The maneuvers should be performed for insertion depths of 6, 5, 4, 3, 2, and 1 cm

8

chapter

2 When squeeze, push/strain, and the rest/relax study is completed for each level, insert the perfused or solid state probe again to a depth of 2–3 cm from the anal verge. Continue the procedure by studying the RAIR and rectal volume sensory thresholds (see numbers 5 & 6, p. 217).

OPTIONAL PROCEDURES

1 Sphincter length

Optionally with the water-perfused or solid state probe the sphincter length can be calculated by performing a stationary/slow pull through or a rapid pull through of the sphincter. The catheter is withdrawn 0.5–1.0 cm each minute to obtain a stationary pull through. Using the rapid pull through the catheter is connected to a puller which automatically withdraws the catheter at a constant speed of 0.5–1.0 cm/s. The HPZ indicates the sphincter length.

2 Vector volume analysis (Fig. 8.77)

The pressure profile of the sphincter can also be studied by using a specific catheter with six to eight radially oriented channels; a so-called "vector volume" catheter. The vector volume analysis can give additional information regarding the geometry of the sphincter. Possible deficiencies and asymmetries are shown on a three-dimensional picture.

Both the SPT technique and rapid pull through technique (by motorized puller) can be used.

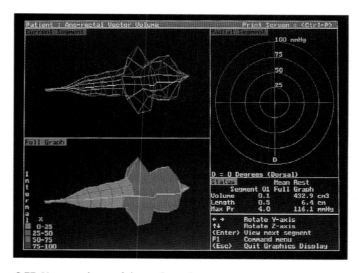

Figure 8.77 Vector volume of the anal canal.

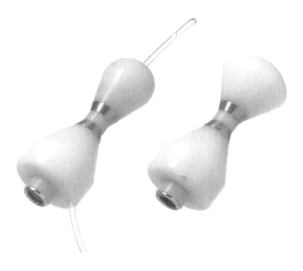

Figure 8.78 Dantec EMG probe for placement in the rectum.

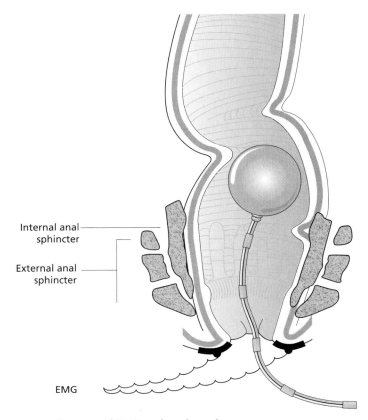

Internal anal
sphincter

External anal
sphincter

EMG

Figure 8.79 Placement of EMG surface electrodes.

chapter 8

3 Defecation dynamics

This can be studied by the following methods:

- Evaluating the combined external and internal anal sphincter pressures, EMG trace, and the abdominal pressure exerted onto the rectum during defecation attempts.

  (a) Position the EMG probe in the rectum. The motility catheter is inserted through the EMG probe's center hole. If external EMG sensors are used instead, two surface electrodes are placed over the external anal sphincter, and the third on the buttocks (Figs 8.78 & 8.79)

  (b) While the patient is lying down ask him/her to strain as if defecating and voluntarily squeeze in a random order

  (c) Normally, during defecation the EMG signal from the external anal sphincter decreases and there is a decrease in anal pressure (Fig. 8.80)

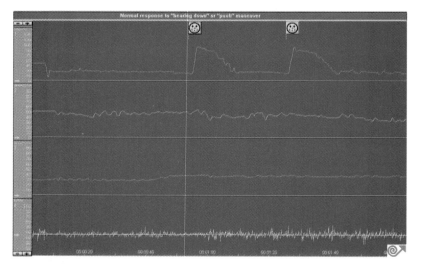

Figure 8.80 Pressure changes in the rectum and anal canal together with the EMG signal from the external anal sphincter during defecation in a healthy individual. There is increased pressure in the rectum, no increase/relaxation of the anal canal and decreased EMG activity.

- Evaluating the ability to defecate a rectal balloon from the rectum. While sitting on a portable toilet stool, the patient should be able to retain and then expel a 150 ml water-filled balloon placed in the rectum
- A synchronized digital imaging system can be used to correlate EMG, sphincter pressures, and defecography in order to study the dynamics of the evacuation process (Fig. 8.81).

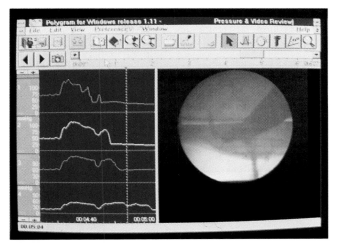

Figure 8.81 Synchronized digital imaging (defecography, motility).

After the study

- Remove the catheter
- Remove EMG probe or surface electrodes if these have been used
- Provide a washcloth and privacy for the patient to get cleaned up
- Patient may resume his/her daily activities
- Record technical observations during the study
- Review the study and generate a report. If desired, print the report
- Clean and disinfect the probes according to hospital regulations and catheter manufacturer's instructions.

Interpretations

The normal RAIR is shown in Fig. 8.82.

MANOMETRIC FINDINGS (Figs 8.83 & 8.84)

Diabetes
- Decrease in rectal sensitivity
- Increased spontaneous sphincter relaxations.

Elderly patients with constipation
- Decreased anal canal resting pressure
- Decreased maximal squeeze pressure.

Anismus (Fig. 8.83)
- Paradoxic contraction of the external anal sphincter and/or puborectalis muscle when the patient strains to defecate
- The rectal threshold volume required to induce an urge to defecate is usually abnormally high.

8

chapter

221

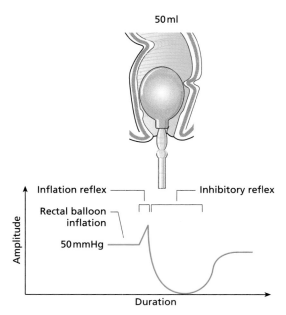

Figure 8.82 Normal RAIR due to distention of the anorectal balloon. Reproduced from Smith LE, *Practical Guide to Anorectal Testing* with permission from Waverly International.

It is important to know that in normal patients anismus may be caused by the embarrassment of defecating while being observed.

Fecal incontinence

There are many different causes of fecal incontinence (see Section 5.4).

On anorectal manometry one can detect several different abnormalities:

- decrease in resting pressure
- decrease in maximum squeeze pressure
- decreased maximum tolerable rectal volume
- reduced rectal volume necessary to induce sphincter relaxation (RAIR)
- impaired external anal sphincter response to rectal distention and increases in intraabdominal pressures (e.g. while coughing)
- impaired sampling function in the anal canal.

A one-page summary report of anorectal manometry is shown in Fig. 8.84.

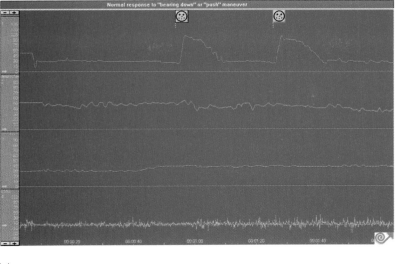

(a)

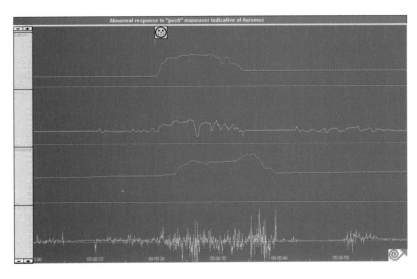

(b)

Figure 8.83 Anorectal manometry showing pressure changes in the rectum and the anal canal together with EMG activity of the external anal sphincter during defecation in (a) a healthy subject and (b) a patient with anismus. In (b) there is a paradoxic increase in pressure and EMG activity of the external sphincter during defecation.

Anorectal Manometry

Patient Name:	**PATIENT, Demo**		
Patient ID #:	123 45 6789		
Referring Physician:	Michaels, J	Physician:	Jones, D
Date of Test:	1996-04-16	Assistant:	

Gastroenterology Dept.
City Hospital

Interpretation and Comments

Procedure consisted of inserting a flexible water perfused catheter into the patients rectum to a depth of 6 cm and withdrawing it in a stepwise fashion; measuring resting and squeeze pressures at 1 cm intervals. The catheter has a latex balloon for distending the rectum located at its distal tip and four radially oriented pressure measuring sites located 7 cm proximal to the balloon.

Rectal Sensation Thresholds

		Normals
First sensation:	30 ml	10 to 30
First urge to defecate:	50 ml	
Maximum tolerable volume:	70 ml	100 to 300

Rectal Compliance Analysis

Units for compliance are : ml/mmHg

		Normals
From 1st sensation to M.T.V.:	3.9	2 to 6

Radial Pressure Analysis

Units: Pressure/Amplitude:mmHg-Rate:mmHg/sec

Resting pressures

cm	Right	Anter.	Left	Post.	HPZ
6	5.2	11.8	12.4	7.0	
5	4.9	11.4	12.9	6.8	
4	22.8	30.8	32.4	35.1	
3	28.6	13.6	19.8	29.3	
2	22.3	14.7	14.1	9.5	
1	9.2	70.8	50.2	18.3	X

Pressure increases during squeeze

cm	Right	Anter.	Left	Post.	HPZ
6	0.0	0.0	22.7	18.1	
5	35.7	41.4	47.4	25.4	
4	20.2	23.3	43.9	31.2	
3	93.5	81.6	49.3	44.3	X
2	62.1	92.5	55.8	42.7	X
1	52.4	86.5	149.8	91.6	X

	Resting	Normals	Squeeze	Normals	Overall
HPZ Length(cm)	1	2.5 to 3.5	3		4
Mean pressure over HPZ	37.1	40 to 70	75.2		90.5
Maximum pressure over HPZ	70.6		149.8	30 to 110	163.6
Verge to maximum (cm)	1		1		1

RectoAnal Inhibitory Reflex (R.A.I.R.)

Present for 30 ml at 3.0 cm from anal verge

Maximum Voluntary Squeeze

Peak amplitude:	57.1
Regression amplitude:	50.0
Duration at 50%	4.3
Fatigue rate:	1.4

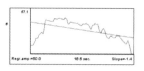

Signature: _____

PW - version 1.11   Anorectal Manometry - version 1.0
Copyright 1995-96, Synectics Medical AB

Michaels, J.   123 45 6789

Figure 8.84 One-page summary report of anorectal manometry (Synectics PW Anorectal Manometry Analysis Module).

8

chapter

8.11 Visceral stimulator/barostat studies

Indications
- To test gastrointestinal muscle tone—gastric fundic motility and rectal/colonic motility
- To test visceral sensory thresholds
- To test visceral compliance.

Equipment
- Visceral stimulator/barostat—a computer-controlled device which makes it possible either to deliver automated, precise stimuli for volume or pressure distention or to keep a constant pressure in the airbag to measure volume variation (guttone) (Fig. 8.85)
- Specific anorectal catheter (visceral stimulator catheter—with air bag and different numbers of perfused ports)
- Analysis software
- Accessories:
  - (a) lubricating gel
  - (b) 4 × 4 gauzes
  - (c) gloves
  - (d) towels and washcloth
  - (e) blue pads.

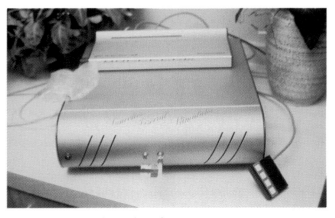

Figure 8.85 Synectics visceral stimulator/barostat.

Before the study
- For rectal testing—bowel cleansing should be limited to a tap water enema to minimize rectal irritation
- For proximal colonic testing—oral colonic lavage is recommended
- For descending colon and sigmoid testing—magnesium citrate enema is recommended

225

- If sedation is needed for colonic probe placement, use 2–5 mg midazolam followed by 0.2–0.4 mg flumazenil to reverse sedation
- Study should be performed in a fasting state due to significant differences in motility and tone between fed and fasting states
- Explain the procedure to the patient to obtain patient cooperation and increase comfort level
- Instruct the patient that the visceral stimulator has a keypad with four keys that he/she can control. The four keybuttons are used for marking sensation, urge, pain, and emergency—the pump immediately withdraws the intraballoon pressure to zero
- Verify signed informed consent (if applicable for the institution)
- Calibrate the equipment according to the user's manual.

Procedure

Three parameters may be studied:
1 muscle tone
2 visceral sensory thresholds
3 visceral compliance.

Patient's position

The position of the patient is of great importance when recording digestive tone from any part of the gut, because the weight of adipose tissue overlying the organ and the tone of the abdominal wall directly influence barostat recordings.

- If colonic/rectal studies are to be performed, the patient should lie on the left side with knees and hips flexed. Insert the probe well lubricated.

  If the probe is to be positioned above the splenic flexure, colonoscopy is needed for placement by directly pulling the probe along with the colonoscope. A guidewire is inserted into the probe to make it more rigid. Anesthesia is required for this placement.

  In colonic studies, the patient is often positioned in a 30° supine position. In rectal studies the patient is positioned in a prone position.
- If gastric studies are to be performed, the patient sits in an upright position during intubation of the catheter through the mouth.

  During the study the patient is then often seated with a 40° incline. Do not let patients have his/her arms crossed over the chest or abdomen

  Allow the patient to get used to the probe. If no air or drugs were used, allow 10–20 min adaptation before testing.

  Wait 1 h before starting the study to allow drug washout and clearance of insufflated air (if probe placement has been performed with colonoscopy).

1 TO EVALUATE MUSCLE TONE
- Find the minimum distending pressure

- The minimal distending pressure is defined as the pressure level that results in a volume greater than 30 ml. The pressure in the patient bag must be greater than the pressure in the organ that is under examination (e.g. intragastric or intrarectal pressures)
- At least 5 (maximum 20) min recording is required to test muscle tone adequately
- Variations of muscle tone can be reported as percentage changes from baseline bag volume.

2 TO EVALUATE ANORECTAL SENSORY THRESHOLDS

- To investigate when and at what level the patient exhibits certain perceived thresholds (e.g. pain, urge to defecate, and the first sensation of defecation)
- Two methods are recommended mainly because they are less vulnerable to psychologic bias.

The tracking technique
- The bag is progressively distended (phasic, stepwise, or ramp distention, see Figs 8.86 & 8.87) until the patient reports pain or other sensations of interest
- Subsequent distentions are then adjusted up or down depending on whether or not the patient reported pain on the previous trial
- If the patient reported pain, the next distention will be decreased or remain the same. If the patient reported no pain, the next distention will be increased or remain the same

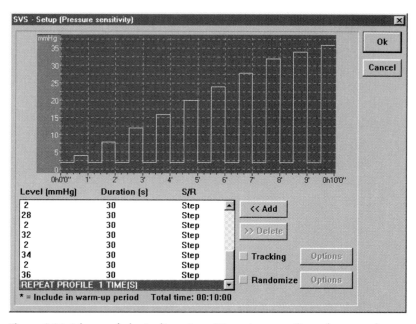

Figure 8.86 Schema of phasic distentions. Distentions are 60 s or longer and separated by intervals of 60 s or longer.

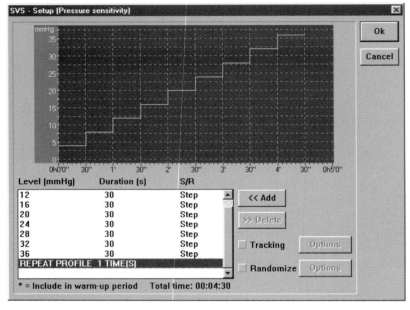

(a)

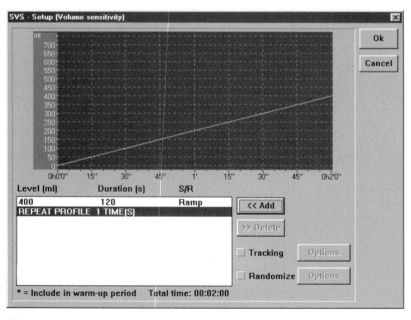

(b)

Figure 8.87 Schema of stepwise and ramp distentions.

- To make the amount of distention unpredictable to the patient, a random numbers algorithm is used to decide whether to decrease the amount of distention or keep it the same following a painful test trial, and similarly to decide whether to increase or keep the distention the same after a non-painful test trial
- Instruct the patient to press the keypad buttons when sensations occur. Pain or other sensations should also be reported on a graduated scale; not only as yes or no
- The threshold is the average intensity over a series of trials for which one tracks (i.e. makes adjustments which are slightly above and below) the threshold
- Sensory thresholds can be reported as bag pressure or bag volume. However, bag pressure is preferable since it is less vulnerable to measurement error.

The double random staircase method (Fig. 8.88)
- The computer starts with a low pressure (e.g. 2 mmHg). If the patient does not report pain, the next stimulus is 2 mmHg higher. The computer then steps rapidly up to the pain threshold. If the patient reports pain, the amount of distention decreases on the next trial. The computer then oscillates around the threshold until the program is stopped. To make the test stimuli unpredictable to the patient, the computer uses two different "staircases." The computer alternates randomly between the two staircases until the patient presses the feedback button three times on each staircase. This means that both the staircases have reached the sensitivity threshold
- The threshold is calculated by taking the average of the pressures associated with the first three positive responses on each staircase.

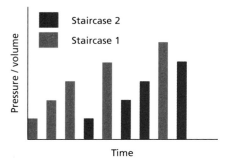

Figure 8.88 Random alteration between the two staircases which makes the test sequence unpredictable to the patient.

3 TO EVALUATE ANORECTAL COMPLIANCE
Compliance of a hollow organ may be defined as the capacity of the organ to adapt to an imposed stretch.

Compliance is defined as the slope of the pressure–volume curve (see Fig. 8.89).

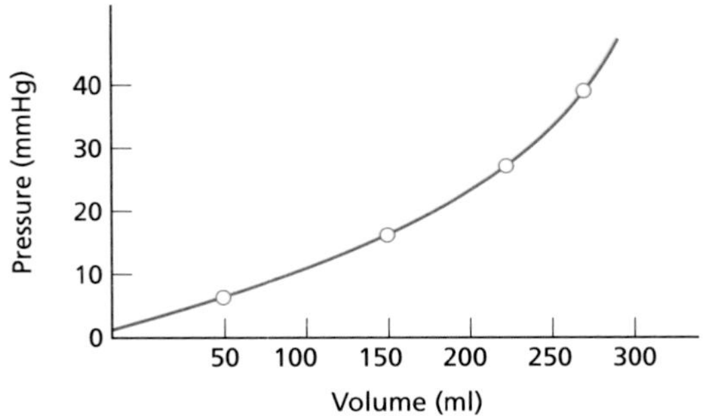

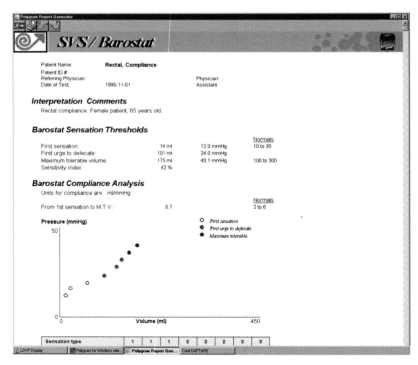

Compliance = ΔV/ΔP

Rectal compliance: $\dfrac{V_2 - V_1}{P_2 - P_1}$

Figure 8.89 Point 1 (P_1, V_1), point 2 (P_2, V_2); compliance $= (V_2 - V_1)/(P_2 - P_1)$.

- Position the visceral stimulator catheter with its infinitely compliant bag in the rectum
- The visceral stimulator/barostat should produce phasic distentions with an increase of 2 mmHg each time until the patient's maximal tolerable volume is reached (Fig. 8.90)

Figure 8.90 The Synectics Barostat Compliance Analysis.

- The compliance is automatically calculated after the set of distentions has been completed. Normal values are usually between 2 and 6 ml/mmHg.

The advantages of using the barostat for rectal compliance measurements are:
- the bag has no compliance in itself compared to the latex/elastic balloons used in traditional anorectal manometry
- the bag is attached at both ends to the catheter which prevents expansion of the bag toward the sigmoid colon
- the barostat makes the procedure much faster and easily reproducible since the protocol is computerized.

After the study
- Remove the catheter
- Provide a washcloth and privacy for the patient to get cleaned up
- Patient may resume his/her daily activities
- Clean the visceral stimulator catheter according to cleaning instructions.

Interpretations
Normal values have not yet been established.
- In some studies an increased sensitivity to anorectal distention has been seen in patients with irritable bowel syndrome
- In patients with megarectum a decreased sensitivity to distention has been seen.

Pitfalls
- Sensory thresholds are higher on rapid inflation than on slow inflation
- Rapid phasic distention may be less physiologic than slow distention.

8

chapter

8.12 Biofeedback

Indications
- Constipation due to ansimus
- Urinary incontinence
- Fecal incontinence due to:
  (a) weak external anal sphincter
  (b) impaired discrimination of rectal sensations
  (c) no synchrony between internal and external anal sphincter response to rectal distention.

Equipment
- Anorectal motility probe with anorectal balloon (perfused or solid state)
- EMG sensors on a rectal probe or external EMG sensors. The advantages of the probe compared to external EMG sensors are that it is easily placed correctly, and it is not sensitive to contractions of the buttocks but provide information about activity of the anus (external sphincter) (see Fig. 8.78)
- Bioamplifier (Fig. 8.91)
- Polygraf
- Pressure transducers
- Personal computer
- Software (anorectal manometry analysis module)
- Accessories:
  (a) examination gloves
  (b) lubricant
  (c) towels and gowns
  (d) 4 × 4 gauze pads.

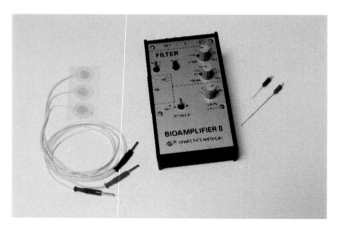

Figure 8.91 The Synectics Bioamplifier II with surface electrodes and needles for recording of EMG activity.

Biofeedback procedure in constipation due to anismus

In patients with anismus (spastic pelvic floor syndrome) there is a paradoxic contraction of the external anal sphincter and/or puborectalis muscle when the patient strains to defecate.

By using biofeedback training with visual feedback, the patient can learn that straining to defecate should be carried out in a different manner, without pelvic floor contraction. The patient can, instead, learn how to relax the external anal sphincter while straining.

1 With the patient in left lateral decubitus position, insert the EMG probe into the rectum (see Fig. 8.78)
2 Insert the anorectal probe through the EMG probe
3 The outputs of the manometric recording and the EMG signals are displayed on the computer
4 The patient lies on his/her side (or in some centers sitting on a commode) and observes the manometric and EMG tracings from a person with normal readings
5 Explain the difference between the healthy person's external sphincter relaxation and the patient's contraction
6 Distend the rectal balloon with 50 ml air or water and ask the patient to push as if defecating
7 While watching his/her own tracings, the patient tries to modify the external sphincter response to make them appear more normal (relaxation of the external anal sphincter)
8 Visual and voice reinforcements are constantly given when correct responses are made
9 The procedure with defecation trials is repeated until the patient is able to relax the external sphincter
10 When the patient is able to relax the external sphincter, he/she is encouraged to do so without rectal balloon distention
11 When the patient manages to relax the external sphincter without balloon distention, the visual and then the verbal feedback is withdrawn.

TRAINING PLAN

A normal biofeedback session lasts approximately 45 min and includes 30–35 defecation trials. One to three sessions per week for 1–6 weeks in a row are usually enough to obtain the goals of biofeedback.

GOAL

When 10 relaxations of the external sphincter can be performed without visual feedback in each of two successive sessions the biofeedback therapy is discontinued.

Biofeedback procedure in fecal incontinence

There are three separate and effective components in the biofeedback training of patients with fecal incontinence:

- training of the external sphincter muscle (in patients with weak anal sphincter)
- training in discrimination of rectal sensations
- training synchrony of the internal and external sphincter responses to rectal distention.

The same set up of the biofeedback procedure is used as in the training of anismus patients.

1 The patient is instructed to focus on sensation in the rectal area
2 Show the patient tracings from a healthy person. Point out the normal external anal sphincter contraction following rectal distention. Instruct the patient to contract the external anal sphincter, including muscles around the anal canal in an attempt to duplicate the tracings from the healthy person. While watching his/her own tracings, the patient tries to modify the external sphincter response making them appear more normal (contraction of the external anal sphincter) (Fig. 8.92)
3 Visual and verbal encouragements are given when the correct responses are performed
4 In order to link external sphincter contraction with rectal distention (and relaxation of the internal sphincter), ask the patient to contract momentarily the external sphincter whenever he/she feels rectal distention. The rectal balloon is inflated until the patient can sense the rectal distention (normally 20–50 ml)
5 After five repetitions of a stimulus at a clearly discernible level (and if the patient has responded to at least three appropriately), the patient is

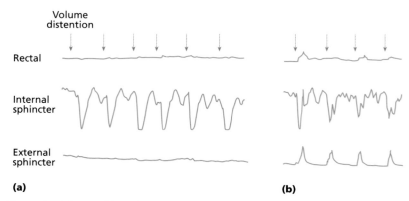

(a)   **(b)**

Figure 8.92 Rectosphincteric responses in an incontinent patient (a) before and (b) after biofeedback training. In (a) there is no contraction of the EAS in response to rectal distention to prevent incontinence. In (b), after biofeedback the EAS contraction in response to rectal distention is achieved.

trained to recognize progressively smaller distention volumes and to synchronize voluntary anal sphincter contraction with the distention

6 Continue decreasing the distention volume until the patient has five successive rectal distentions to which there is no response. Then go back to the distention volume above the unresponsive distentions, and continue the training at this level (at least two series of five distentions). After this, try to lower the distention again. It will help the patient focus on the sensation at the threshold level, and possibly lower their sensation threshold

7 Approximately 50 training trials in total are performed in each session

8 Encourage the patient to increase the amplitude and duration of the voluntary anal sphincter squeeze.

GOAL

Rectal sensation thresholds are often lowered and sphincter contractile responses restored after only a few biofeedback training sessions.

Normally, biofeedback training is discontinued after three to five training sessions.

There are instruments for home biofeedback training which can be very useful to some patients. The patient should practice anal sphincter and pelvic floor contraction at least every other day for 20–30 min.

chapter 8

8.13 Pudendal nerve terminal motor latency test

The function of the pudendal nerve can be tested by transrectally stimulating the motor nerve electrically and measuring the time taken from stimulation to the first measurable contraction of the external anal sphincter.

Indications
- To investigate if pudendal neuropathy is the cause of disorders such as:
  (a) fecal incontinence
  (b) perineal descent syndrome
  (c) urethral incontinence—to assess indirectly perineal nerve dysfunction (one branch of the pudendal nerve, the perineal nerve, innervates the periurethral striated muscle)
- Pre- or postsurgical evaluation of sphincter reconstructions (e.g. after damage related to vaginal delivery) or rectal prolapse repairs
- In patients with long-term problems of constipation and straining prior to rectal resection in order to predict the likelihood of incontinence. Repeated straining of stool with traction of the pelvic floor may lead to stretch-induced injury to the pudendal nerve.

Contraindications
- Uncooperative patient
- Acute inflammation/infection of the rectal mucosa, anal canal, or the perineum
- Anal stenosis.

Equipment
- Disposable pudendal nerve stimulating and recording device (e.g. Medtronic–Dantec St Mark's electrode) (Fig. 8.93)
- Combined EMG and nerve conduction velocity testing equipment (e.g. Medtronic–Dantec, Cantata, Keypoint or Keypoint portable)
- Ground electrode (a saline-soaked contact band connected to the equipment)
- Water-soluble lubricant
- Surgical gloves
- Blue pads
- Towels and washcloth.

Before the study
- In some centers the patient is given a small enema
- No sedation is given to the patient
- Explain the procedure to the patient
- Written consent is signed if the institution requires it.

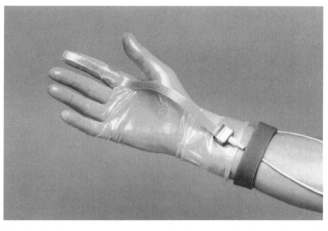

Figure 8.93 St Mark's electrode consists of a bipolar stimulating electrode, which should be mounted on the tip of the finger, and recording electrodes which detect contraction responses of the external anal sphincter located 3 cm proximal to the base of the finger.

Procedure

1 Patient should be positioned on his/her left side, with hips and knees flexed. Place a blue pad under the buttocks
2 The examiner puts on surgical gloves. The talc is washed off the gloves and they are then carefully dried. The saline soaked grounding electrode strap is mounted on the examiner's wrist around the electrode lead and then the St Mark's pudendal electrode is mounted on the index finger
3 Connect the stimulating electrodes to the stimulating source of the EMG and nerve conduction velocity testing equipment and the recording electrodes to the recording input channel on the equipment
4 Coat the electrodes with electrode gel
5 To facilitate insertion of the finger into the rectum, place a small amount of water-soluble lubricant at the tip of the finger (on the side opposite the electrode). Too much gel could result in a bad recording as it may short circuit the electrodes. To avoid artifactual recordings secondary to grounding, the lubricant must be prevented from entering the outer glove
6 Insert the finger into the rectum and palpate the left and right ischial spine (just above the pelvic floor)—the site where the pudendal nerve leaves the pelvis through the greater sciatic notch (Fig. 8.94)
7 Stimulate the pudendal nerve on the left side, and note the contraction of the external anal sphincter. Press with the finger to get both stimulation points in contact with the pudendal nerve. Move the tip of the finger slowly across the pelvic wall and note the maximal response over the nerve. The latency of the response is visualized on the screen of the EMG and nerve conduction velocity testing equipment

8

chapter

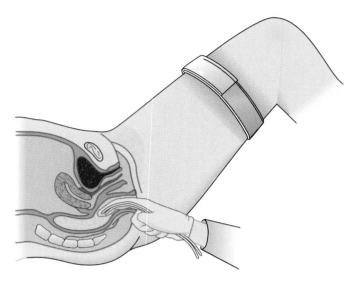

Figure 8.94 Use of the St Mark's pudendal electrode. Insert the index finger mounted with the electrode into the rectum and palpate the left and right ischial spines. The pudendal nerve is then stimulated at these sites.

8 The right pudendal nerve is then studied. Occasionally the patient may need to be repositioned in the right lateral decubitus position in order to find the maximal response to stimulation of the right pudendal nerve.

After the study
- Provide a washcloth and give the patient privacy to get cleaned up
- Patient may resume his/her daily activities
- Record technical observations.

Interpretations
- The terminal motor latency is the measurement of the fastest response in the pudendal nerve–external sphincter mechanism. The latency of response is measured from the onset of the stimulus to the response with external anal sphincter contraction (Fig. 8.95)
- The normal values for pudendal nerve terminal motor latency have been shown to be 2.0 ± 0.2 msec
- The right and left pudendal nerve latencies may be different, but should differ only slightly from the mean
- Patients with idiopathic fecal incontinence and patients with perineal descent have often been found to have prolonged pudendal nerve terminal latencies

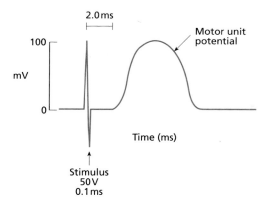

Figure 8.95 Terminal motor latency.

- Note:
  - (a) normal latency does not indicate absence of nerve damage
  - (b) abnormal latency does not indicate abnormal muscle function
  - (c) single fiber EMG is necessary to quantitate damage.

8.14 Sphincter of Oddi manometry

Indications

- *Type I*: in patients that have biliary-type pain and *one or two* of the following objective criteria:

  (a) elevated liver function tests (should be documented on two or more occasions)

  (b) dilatation of the common bile duct (over 12 mm), or

  (c) delayed contrast drainage (over 45 min) of contrast from the common bile duct during endoscopic retrograde cholangiopancreatographic (ERCP) study

- *Type II*: prepapillotomy. If one or two of the criteria above exist, sphincter of Oddi manometry is useful to decide if papillotomy should be performed. If all three criteria exist, manometry is not necessary prior to endoscopic or operative ablation of the distal choledochal sphincter

- *Type III*: in patients with biliary-type pain (but no objective finding supportive of biliary tract obstruction), sphincter of Oddi manometry may be considered after careful clinical assessment and exclusion of irritable bowel syndrome

(*Type I–III* are classified according to the standard criteria defined by Genen)

- Patients with recurrent pancreatitis or pancreatic pain without organic disease
- Patients with chronic pancreatitis
- Patients with common bile duct stones.

Contraindications

- Inexperienced endoscopist. The endoscopist has to be experienced in cannulating the appropriate ductal system. In addition, training is required to be able to recognize an acceptable sphincter of Oddi recording and interpret it appropriately
- Significant bleeding diathesis.

Complications

- There is a significant risk of pancreatitis following sphincter of Oddi manometry. Complications increase if:

  (a) the pancreatic duct is cannulated and the pressure in the pancreatic duct segment of the sphincter of Oddi is recorded

  (b) if a water-perfused system, without aspiration, is used

- Cholangitis
- Duodenal perforation (rare)
- Hemorrhage (rare)
- Hyperamylasemia without clinical pancreatitis is commonly seen.

Equipment

- Sphincter of Oddi solid state motility catheter (one channel) or perfused

one or three lumen motility catheter (1.7 mm) with or without aspiration port
- Hydraulic perfusion system—infusion rate 0.12–0.25 ml/min (sterile water). Since sphincter of Oddi manometry must be a sterile procedure, remember to sterilize the container and capillaries
- Polygraf
- Personal computer
- Software
- Endoscope (duodenoscope)
- Guidewire (optional)
- Anesthetic spray (e.g. Lidocaine)
- Needles
- Sedatives (midazolam or diazepam)
- Cholecystokinin (CCK for IV administration)
- For ERCP
  (a) cannulas filled with renografin diluted to 30%
  (b) fluoroscope with spot film cassettes
  (c) lead aprons and thyroid collars
- 4 × 4 gauze
- Gloves
- Towels and washcloth.

Before the study
- Patient should come to the laboratory after an overnight fast (6–8 h of fasting) to prevent aspiration during intubation
- Verify signed informed consent (if needed for the institution)
- Explain the procedure to the patient to obtain patient cooperation
- Sedation is given to the patient prior to the study. Sedation has not been proven to change sphincter of Oddi motility. Anesthetize the patient's throat with a topical agent. Administer midazolam or diazepam IV until an appropriate level of sedation is reached
- All personnel must wear lead aprons and thyroid collars if ERCP spot filming is to be performed
- Calibrate catheter according to manufacturer's instructions.

Procedure
With sphincter of Oddi manometry (Fig. 8.96) the following parameters should be recorded:
- common bile duct pressure
- basal sphincter of Oddi pressure
- phasic wave pressure
- duodenal pressure

Procedure is as follows:
1 Position the patient on his/her left side with left arm behind the back to

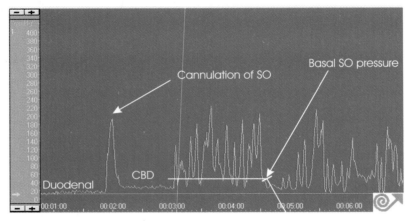

Figure 8.96 Station pull through of the sphincter of Oddi (SO). The tracing shows the duodenal baseline, the pressure rise when cannulating the SO to position the catheter in the common bile duct (CBD) and the slow pull through of the SO. The basal pressure of the recorded sphincter is approximately 30 mmHg.

facilitate the roll to the prone position required for cannulation and spot filming

2 Intubate duodenoscope and localize the papilla Vater

3 One of two methods may be used to position the motility catheter:

(a) Cannulate the sphincter of Oddi with the ERCP catheter. Normally contrast is inserted to visualize the biliary tree and determine the catheter's placement in the common bile duct. Insert a guidewire of at least 300 cm in length through the ERCP catheter. Withdraw the ERCP catheter and slide the manometry catheter over the guidewire. Once the manometry catheter is in place, remove the guidewire

(b) Position the manometry catheter by passing it through the biopsy channel of a side viewing duodenoscope, manipulating it through the papilla into the common bile duct. Catheter position can be verified by using a small amount of contrast injected through the catheter lumen

4 Wait a few minutes before starting the procedure to avoid artifacts

5 Record the common bile duct pressure for a few minutes until a stable baseline pressure is obtained

6 Withdraw catheter slowly in 2-mm increments at 2-min intervals (SPT). An HPZ is encountered as the catheter is withdrawn. When all three ports are located within the HPZ record the basal sphincter pressure for at least 3–5 min

7 Note phasic wave propagation (phasic waves are superimposed on the basal pressure) and the amplitude, frequency, and duration of the waves

8 Continue withdrawal of the catheter. When the recording channels reach

chapter 8

the duodenum, the pressure falls below the pressure in the common bile duct. Duodenal pressure is measured

9 If necessary repeat the SPT of the sphincter of Oddi

10 CCK may be administered intravenously to the patient. In a healthy person, this would lead to a decrease in the frequency and amplitude of phasic waves and to a decrease in the basal sphincter of Oddi pressure.

After the study

- Remove the manometry catheter
- Monitor patient's vital signs
- Let the patient stay and rest at the hospital for a while, mainly to let sedation wear off
- Do not give the patient anything orally until the gag reflex and sensation in the throat return
- Remove the IV line
- Patient should not drive for 6–8 h after conscious sedation
- Give patient written instructions. Many patients do not recall verbal instructions after sedation
- Only clear liquids are permitted for 24 h after the pharyngeal function has returned
- Clean and disinfect the catheter according to hospital regulations and catheter manufacturer's instructions
- Interpret data from recording.

Interpretations

NORMAL VALUES

- Basal sphincter of Oddi pressure: 10–20 mmHg (values are calculated with the duodenal baseline used as the zero reference)
- Phasic wave amplitude: 100–140 mmHg
- Phasic wave frequency: 3–6 waves/min
- Retrograde contractions 5–20%.

MANOMETRIC FINDINGS DURING SPHINCTER OF ODDI DYSMOTILITY

(Figs 8.97 & 8.98)

- Elevated basal sphincter of Oddi pressure—more than 40 mmHg above the duodenal pressure
- An increased choledochoduodenal pressure gradient
- High frequency of contractions—greater than 10 waves/min
- Predominance of retrograde propagating waves (over 50% of the time)
- Paradoxic increase in sphincter pressure in response to CCK
- Increased amplitude of phasic contractions—greater than 200–300 mmHg.

Of these, an elevated basal pressure is the most discriminatory; the relative importance of these other criteria has not been defined.

chapter 8

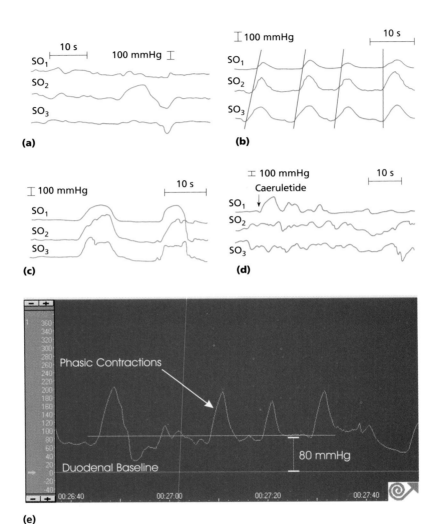

Figure 8.97 Examples of manometric findings in sphincter of Oddi (SO) dyskinesia. (a) Increased SO baseline pressure and dyscoordinated waves; (b) retrograde SO phasic waves; (c) increased phasic wave amplitude; (d) absent inhibition of SO activity following Caeruletide, and (e) tracing showing a basal SO pressure of 80 mmHg. Superimposed on this basal level are seen SO contractions. (a)–(d) Reproduced from Funch-Jensen P. Sphincter of Oddi Motility. *Acta Chirug Scand.* 1990; Suppl. 553, with permission from Almqvist & Wiksell.

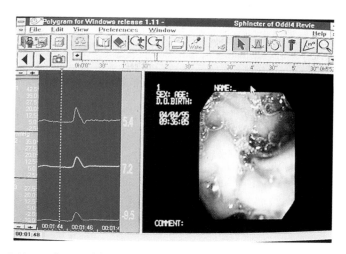

Figure 8.98 Synchronized biliary video manometry.

Pitfalls

- Directly after cannulation there is an initial hyperactivity. To avoid this, keep the catheter still for a few minutes before starting the recording
- Any intraabdominal pressure rise (such as retching, valsalva, hyperventilation, etc.) will be transmitted to the measuring system and cause artifacts
- Catheter movement may give rise to reading errors.

9 Clinical Procedures in Children

9.1 24-h pH-metry

Indications

- The diagnosis and treatment of gastroesophageal reflux (GER). The investigation will be of value if the result will change the management of the child with regards to regurgitation and vomiting. If esophagitis has already been diagnosed with endoscopy or biopsy, there is no need for pH-metry to document the presence of gastroesophageal reflux disease (GERD)
- Patients with unusual presentations of GERD (e.g. laryngeal symptoms, atypical chest pain, recurrent pneumonia, apnea, reactive airways disease, dystonia)
- Pre- and posttreatment evaluation (e.g. to evaluate if the dosage of medication is optimal)
- Pre- and postantireflux surgery
- Research.

Equipment (Fig. 9.1)

- pH catheter

  (a) it is preferable to use a catheter with as small a diameter as possible to avoid influencing the esophageal function in the child and to avoid hypersalivation. A catheter with a diameter that is too large may cause repetitive swallowing which induces primary esophageal peristalsis and may normalize pH monitoring due to better esophageal clearance

  (b) catheter—glass microelectrodes (approximately 1.5 mm) with external reference, or

  (c) disposable antimony catheter with internal reference (approximately 2.3 mm in diameter), or

  (d) multiuse antimony catheter with external reference (approximately 1.5 mm in diameter). Only for use in premature babies, since these are too flexible in older babies

- The rest of the equipment needed is the same as in adult pH-metry (see Section 8.2).

Before the study

- No special patient preparation is needed

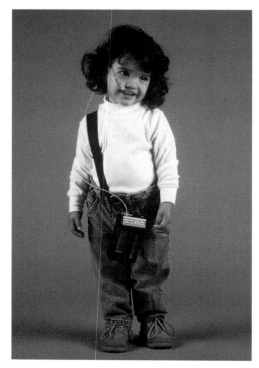

Figure 9.1 Child with pH equipment.

- Avoid introducing the catheter in the postprandial period to avoid nausea, vomiting, and aspiration. If possible, have the child fast for 3–6 h before the study
- Discontinue all antireflux medication 24–48 h prior to the study:
  (a) omeprazole should be avoided 7 days prior to the study
  (b) prokinetics should be avoided 48 h before the pH monitoring
- Assess patient information from parents:
  (a) medical history
  (b) symptoms
  (c) medications
  (d) allergies
- Explain the procedure to the child (if the child is old enough) and the parents to obtain patient cooperation and increase comfort level
- Verify signed informed consent (if applicable for the institution).

During study

Activities
Normal.

Diet

Most centers instruct the patient to continue his/her normal diet so that the study does not alter the daily habits. However, some centers instruct the patient to avoid intake of acid foods and drinks (carbonated beverages, tea, fruit juice, tomatoes, or candy) during the study. Other instructions include:

(a) no chewing gum

(b) no gastric acid reduction medications, laxatives, antacids, or non-steroidals should be taken during testing period

(c) very hot beverages and chilled food (e.g. ice-cream) should be forbidden since electrodes are temperature sensitive.

Position of child

There are varying opinions regarding the optimal position of small children and infants. Crying time, which should be minimized preferably, is often decreased in a prone position. However, there are fewer normal reflux episodes to study lying down. If the child is in a sitting position, there is more acid reflux than when lying down due to the increased intraabdominal pressure. This position may not, however, be as comfortable for the infant. Older children can "live normally" just as in adult pH-metry.

Event buttons

If possible, instruct the child and the parents on how to operate the event buttons in the pH recorder during the study. The buttons on the pH recorder are used to mark different periods and events. Examples of event buttons are given below:

 Chest pain/heartburn

 Meals/eating

 Recumbent/sleep

 Experience different user-defined symptoms like belching, hiccupping, vomiting or coughing

Diary

Instruct the parents to keep a diary during the study to record meals, sleep, and symptoms noting their time of occurrence using the time displayed on the pH recorder.

Procedure

Several methods can be used to position the catheter electrode, such as fluoroscopy, the method recommended by the European Society for Pediatric Gastroenterology and Nutrition (ESPGAN) working group on GER. The catheter should be positioned so that it overlies the third vertebral body, above the diaphragm through'out the respiration cycle.

In children younger than 1 year, Strobel's formula may be used to calculate the approximate length of the esophagus to the lower esophageal sphincter (LES) (from nares to LES). The equation is:

The length of the esophagus to the LES

= the length of the child × 0.252 + 5

The pH sensor should then be positioned at 87% of the esophageal length

- Manometry is ideal for defining catheter placement, but is invasive and time-consuming
- Endoscopy.

Remember that if a catheter with an external reference is used, the reference may be placed on the back of the child to avoid the child touching and moving the reference.

The pH study should be performed the same as in adults (see Section 8.2).

After the study

The child can resume his/her normal activities and diet, and recommence any discontinued medications.

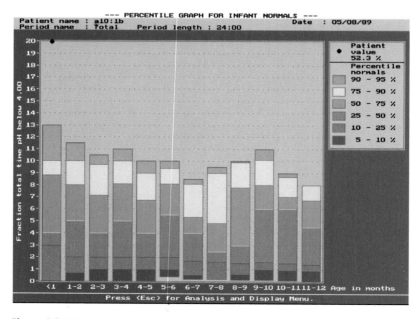

Figure 9.2 ESPGAN scores.

Interpretations

The same parameters are sought as in adults.

To simplify the diagnosis of pathologic reflux in children, the Boix–Ochoa score or the Vandenplas (ESPGAN) scores may be used.

The Boix–Ochoa score is basically the DeMeester and Johnson score (see p. 149) adapted for use in infants. In addition to the total, upright, and supine periods, the pH recording is also studied for the time in which the child is in the prone position.

The ESPGAN score also takes the normal reflux index according to age distribution into consideration (Fig. 9.2).

The total acid exposure time (reflux index) is regarded by some investigators as the most important variable in clinical practice.

Normals

In children, 0–12 months old, the fraction time (RI) (i.e. the percentage of time pH is below 4) should not be above 10% (Fig. 9.3).

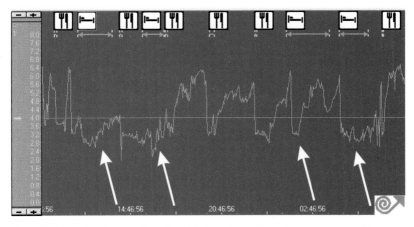

Figure 9.3 Tracing from a 5-week-old infant, born 7 weeks premature, with symptoms of apnea, bradycardia and failure to thrive. 24-h pH monitoring showed increased acid exposure especially during supine position. Reflux index/fraction time 52% (normal 13%, according to ESPGAN scores). Arrows show reflux (pH < 4) during supine position.

9

chapter

9.2 Stationary esophageal manometry

Indications
- To define esophageal motility disorders (e.g. achalasia)
- Pre- and postantireflux surgery
- To evaluate the results of medical and surgical treatments
- Determination of LES prior to 24-h pH-metry
- To evaluate the pathophysiologic mechanism underlying GER-associated diseases.

Contraindications
- See contraindications for nasal intubation (see Section 7.2)
- Patients with cardiac instability or other conditions in whom vagal stimulation is poorly tolerated.

Equipment
- Water-perfused multilumen (four channels) catheter, 3 mm or less in diameter, with side holes 3 cm apart oriented radially at 90° angles or solid state catheter.
- If water-perfused catheter is to be used, a hydraulic capillary infusion system is needed. In small children, the infusion rate must be reduced compared to adults (0.1–0.25 ml/min).

The rest of the equipment needed is the same as in adult esophageal manometry (see Section 8.4).

Before the study
- Assess patient information:
  (a) medical history
  (b) symptoms
  (c) medications
  (d) allergies
- Verify signed informed consent from parents (if applicable for the institution)
- If possible, all medications that could interfere with the motility study should stop 48 h prior to the study. H_2-receptor antagonists should be stopped 3–4 days before pH-monitoring
- Patient should fast for 3–5 h before the study, depending on age
- Patients less than 5 years old should be awakened early in the morning, at least 5–6 h before the study, so that they may nap spontaneously during the study
- If possible, it is important to explain to the child that the passage of the tube through the throat may be uncomfortable, but that it will feel better after the first few swallows. Also, explain the rest of the procedure to increase patient cooperation and comfort level
- Sedation should not be given routinely. It may interfere with swallowing and influence pressures.

Procedure

The procedure is performed the same as in adults with only a few differences (see Section 8.4).

1 The withdrawal of the catheter should be performed in 0.5-cm steps instead of 1-cm steps
2 To perform wet swallows, give the patient 1–2 ml of water from a syringe
3 If patient is older than 3 years, ask the patient to swallow
4 If the child is very young or if there is an uncooperative child, water can be inserted in the mouth while he/she is using a pacifier. The child can be triggered to swallow by moving the pacifier in the mouth
5 If the child does not swallow within 20 s, give another sip of water
6 Provocative testing, "Bernstein test," can be performed at the end of the motility study. 0.1 N HCl is perfused for 5–15 min to reproduce symptoms associated with GER.

Interpretation

It is difficult to recruit normal children for manometric studies (Fig. 9.4). Due to lack of available normal data, normals vary slightly between different

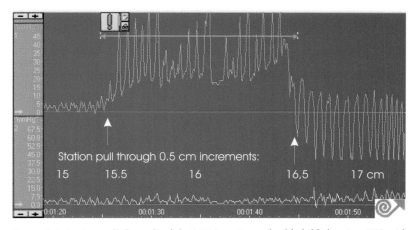

Figure 9.4 Station pull through of the LES in a 9-month-old child showing LES with a length of 1 cm.

Table 9.1 Normal values for esophageal manometry in children.

	Cucchiara et al. (1985) n = 16 Mean age = 11 months	Mahony et al. (1988) n = 9 Age range = 3 months–2 years
Amplitude (mmHg)	59 ± 20	72 ± 17.2
Duration (sec)	2.4 ± 0.2	3.9 ± 1.0
Velocity (cm/s)	3 ± 0.9	2.9 ± 2.1
LES basal pressure (mmHg)	15 ± 2	21.9

LES, lower esophageal sphincter.

laboratories. Variability is also attributable to differences in technique and methods. However, some control data have been published (Table 9.1).

Manometric findings

ACHALASIA (Figs 9.5 & 9.6)

- Incomplete LES relaxation
- Hypertensive basal LES pressure

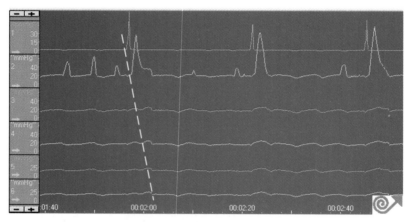

Figure 9.5 Tracing from a 10-year-old child with achalasia. The two proximal channels show normal peristaltic contractions of the striated muscles in the pharynx and the proximal esophagus, whereas the four distal channels show absent esophageal peristalsis. Please also observe the elevated esophageal baseline often seen in patients with achalasia. The cursor shows absence of the contractions in the lower two-thirds of the esophagus where the smooth muscle dominates.

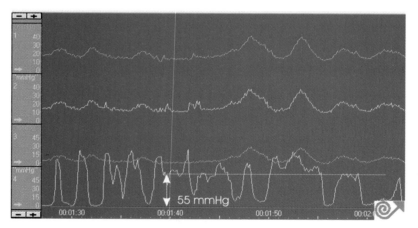

Figure 9.6 Achalasia in a 10-year-old child. Station pull through of the LES shows a hypertensive LES with maximum end-expiratory pressure of 55 mmHg. Red horizontal line shows end-expiratory gastric baseline.

- Absence of esophageal body peristalsis
- Elevated intraesophageal pressure.

SCLERODERMA

- Low or absent LES pressure
- Weak or absent distal esophageal peristalsis
- Weak or distal esophageal contractions and peristalsis
- Normal upper esophageal peristalsis and upper esophageal sphincter (UES).

DERMATOMYOSITIS/POLYMYOSITIS (Fig. 9.7)

- Normal LES pressure and relaxation
- Normal peristalsis in the distal esophageal body
- A decrease in the amplitude of the contraction waves in the proximal esophagus
- An increase in the number of swallows followed by simultaneous waves in the proximal esophagus.

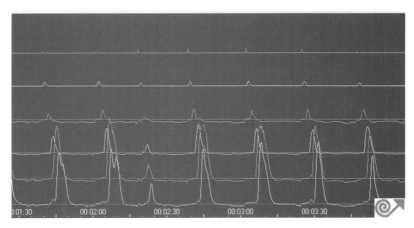

Figure 9.7 Esophageal manometry in a 13-year-old girl with dermatomyositis. There is poor contractile activity in the proximal channels (pharynx and upper esophagus) where the striated muscle fibers are affected by the disease.

MIXED CONNECTIVE TISSUE DISEASE

Esophageal manometric findings similar to scleroderma
- decrease in LES pressure
- decrease in distal esophageal peristalsis.

NEUROLOGIC DISEASES

- Decreased amplitude of the esophageal waves
- Abnormal motor response.

9.3 Antroduodenal manometry

Indications

- Chronic intestinal pseudoobstruction (CIP)
- Predictions of drug effect—the acute effect of prokinetic drugs (cisapride, metoclopramide, domperidone, erythromycin, and somatostatin) can be ascertained during motility tests. Some manometric findings such as the presence of a migrating motor complex (MMC) predicts a good response of cisapride without the need of provocation testing
- In patients with systemic diseases that may affect gastrointestinal motility (e.g. diabetes mellitus and progressive systemic sclerosis)
- In preterm infants to predict feeding intolerance. If an infant's motility index increases after a test feeding, it is likely to tolerate enteral feeding
- In patients with CIP to predict if they are likely to tolerate jejunal feeding. Patients with MMCs are more likely to tolerate this than those without MMCs.

Before the study

- Assess patient information:
  - (a) medical history
  - (b) symptoms
  - (c) medications
  - (d) allergies
- Verify signed informed consent from parents (if applicable for the institution)
- If possible, stop all medication that could interfere with the motility study 48 h prior to the study
- Patient should fast for 3–5 h before the study, depending on age
- Patients less than 5 years old should be awakened early in the morning, at least 5–6 h before the study, so that they may nap spontaneously during the procedure
- If possible, it is important to explain to the child that the passage of the tube through the throat may be uncomfortable, but that it will feel better after the first few swallows. In addition, explain the rest of the procedure to obtain patient cooperation and increase comfort level
- Sedation should not be given routinely.

Equipment

- Catheter: must be soft and thin (less than 2 mm in diameter in infants younger than 6 months). If the catheter is too thick, it may partially obstruct the pylorus slowing gastric emptying. If the catheter is too stiff, it may cause duodenal perforation which has been reported in rare cases during duodenal tube alimentation. In motility testing of infants, solid state catheters are usually too hard and are not appropriate

- Normal configuration of the catheter is at least three sensors. This is sufficient to determine MMC. For antroduodenal manometry one or two recording sites are located in the antrum and the remainder in the duodenum. Distances between recording sites must be based on the purpose of the test
- If a water-perfused system is used in infants, the volume of infused water must be calculated to avoid overhydration or electrolyte imbalance
- The infusion rate must be reduced for small children.

Procedure

Three factors are important to study during the procedure:
- frequency and morphology of MMCs
- propagation velocity of MMCs
- the interruption of MMC activity, and the induction of a fed response following an appropriate meal.

Methods used for placement of the catheter are as follows:

1 Fluoroscopy is commonly used for tube placement. Transpyloric passage may be difficult if a soft tube is used. If a stiff tube is used, transpyloric passage may be easier; but the advancement through the duodenal bulb may be more difficult because of the acute angulations. A weighted metal tip may help guide the catheter by gravity. A small balloon at the tip of the catheter, which is inflated in the duodenum, may also guide the catheter. Some centers use prokinetic drugs (erythromycin or metoclopramide) to increase gastric motility and advance the tube. In this case, the actual study should not be performed until the day after catheter insertion to avoid acute motility effects of these drugs

2 Endoscopy may also be used to position the tube. As little air as possible must be delivered, since distention of the intestinal wall affects motility

3 Direct catheter placement in infants can be achieved without fluoroscopic guidance. The catheter is inserted from the nose to the stomach in a fasting baby. The catheter is then advanced less than 0.1 cm/min. When bile exits from the tube or when the typical duodenal clusters of contractions are recorded, the tube is judged to be in the duodenum.

Recordings should be obtained for at least 3–4 h to determine the presence of phase 3. Provocation with infusion of erythromycin may be used. Intravenous erythromycin induces phase 3 in healthy subjects. Postprandial motility should also be evaluated. A meal inhibits the MMC and induces postprandial motility patterns.

Interpretations

- Premature infants (less than 32 weeks of postconceptional age) do not have an MMC pattern
- Phase 3 in infants differs from adults and is dependent on postconceptional age. By 40 weeks' gestation the pattern is qualitatively similar to adults. In

9

chapter

preterm infants migration velocity is slower, mean interval between phase 3 episodes is shorter, and peak amplitude of contractions is less
- Clustered contractions occurring in the antrum and the duodenum are the dominant motility pattern in fasting and fed infants. From 32 to 40 weeks' gestation these contractions have the same frequency as phase 3, but do not migrate caudally.

It is unknown at what age these clusters disappear, but in adults they are absent or comprise less than 10% of total phase 2 recording time. In certain motility disorders in adults (such as mechanical obstruction, diabetic gastroparesis, and CIP), these clusters may dominate in phase 2.

In visceral myopathies
The phasic pressure waves of the MMC are of low amplitude or do not exist at all.

In visceral neuropathies
There are four abnormal contraction patterns that may occur either by themselves or in various combinations:
- abnormal configuration and propagation of the MMC
- uncoordinated bursts of phasic pressure activity
- uncoordinated intestinal pressure activity that lasts for more than 30 min
- failure of a meal to induce a fed pattern.

Pitfalls
The effect of intravenous infusions must be taken into account. High blood glucose levels (higher than 140 mg/dl) reduce the occurrence of gastric phase 3. Also hyperglycemia inhibits gastric emptying.

9.4 Colonic manometry

Indications
- In constipated children to differentiate between neuropathy or myopathy
- Prior to colectomy (e.g. a child with pseudoobstruction and normal colonic motility does not benefit from total colectomy)
- Preoperatively to decide whether or not to reconnect a diverted colon (e.g. in a child with colonic pseudoobstruction where ileostomy has been made).

Equipment
- Catheter: water-perfused or solid state catheter. Catheter to the visceral stimulator/barostat if this is to be used (SVS catheter)
- Configuration of catheter: distance between recording sites varies from 5 to 15 cm. 15 cm spacing may be used if the catheter can be advanced more than 60 cm from the anus. However, at these intervals contractions that occur between the recording sites may be missed. Traditional motility catheters (solid state and water perfused) may underestimate the true contractile activity within the bowel wall. They only record contractions that occlude the lumen or squeeze a confined region with sufficient force to increase the intraluminal pressure
- SVS catheter. The barostat, with its inflated bag, can measure the true activity in a hollow organ such as the colon. However, it has not been clarified whether it may cause artifacts due to distention of the wall and to obstructing the movement of feces. The SVS is still mainly used in research
- Polygraf or visceral stimulator/barostat
- Personal computer
- Analysis software
- Lubricating gel
- 4 × 4 gauze
- Gloves
- Towels and washcloth
- Three-way stopcocks.

Before the study
- Diet: liquid diet 48 h prior to the study. Standard, balanced oral electrolyte solution on the day before the study
- Enemas should be avoided since they increase colonic contractile activity
- Sedation: children require sedation during placement of the catheter. Avoid narcotics which decrease gastrointestinal activity. Short-acting benzodiazepines are recommended
- If the patient requires deeper sedation and is asleep, leave the catheter in place and perform the procedure the following day.

Procedure

PLACEMENT OF CATHETER

1 Colonoscopy is used for placement of the tip of the catheter. When the colonoscope is advanced beyond the splenic flexure, the guidewire, which has a diameter of 0.052 cm and a soft tip (to minimize the risk of trauma), is passed through the endoscope. The endoscope is then withdrawn, and the motility catheter is placed over the guidewire. The guidewire is removed once the motility catheter is in place. Tape the catheter securely to the patient's buttocks

2 It is important to aspirate air when removing the endoscope since distention from air can cause motility abnormalities

3 If the SVS catheter is to be used, the above procedure to place the catheter cannot be used since the central lumen is closed at the tip (to make it possible to inflate the balloon). The guidewire can instead be inserted into the catheter to make it stiffer and the SVS catheter is then positioned through the colonoscope (see Fig. 8.85)

4 Confirm the catheter's placement by fluoroscopy or radionuclide imaging (infuse a radionuclide marker mixed with a small amount of water through each recording site)

5 It is easier to visualize the catheter on X-rays if the guidewire is left *in situ*. It can then be removed under fluoroscopic control to verify that the catheter remains in position.

DURING THE STUDY

1 When the child recovers from sedation, colonic manometry can be initiated

2 The person that has already met the child, explained the procedure, and taken care of him/her before the study, should be present during the study to reduce the child's anxiety

3 Parents should be encouraged to stay with the child during the procedure. Ask them to bring toys and food with them to distract the child. Since movements and crying create artifacts during the recording, videotapes and games may also be useful in keeping the child still; however, talking, laughing, and eating (after the first hour of fasting) during the study, is allowed.

MANOMETRY

1 Motility while fasting is recorded for 1 h

2 If water-perfused catheters are used, an infusion rate of 10 ml/h is enough to avoid occlusion of the catheter's orifices by stool

3 Give the child a meal, and continue to record normally for another 3 h. Note if there is a gastrocolonic response to the meal (increased motility)

4 If the child falls asleep, observe if motility increases upon awakening.

Provocative testing

Bisacodyl stimulation test—0.2 mg/kg bisacodyl diluted in 5 ml 0.9% NaCl is given as an infusion through the manometry catheter into the transverse colon. In children with normal motility, this induces high-amplitude peristaltic contractions (HAPC).

Interpretations

- Myopathies: no colonic contractions are found
- Neuropathies: contractions are present but uncoordinated
- Normal colonic motility: presence of HAPC, gastrocolonic response and absence of abnormal features (Fig. 9.8).

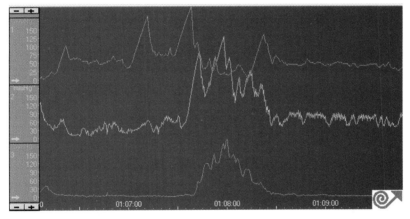

Figure 9.8 Propagating mass movement in the colon. The tracing shows a large pressure wave propagating through the transverse colon.

Pitfalls

- A partly coiled catheter may record contractions that seem to have both oral and aboral migration
- A completely coiled catheter in a dilated rectum only shows simultaneous low-amplitude contractions
- If the child falls asleep immediately after feeding, the gastrocolonic response will not occur. Keep the child awake if possible
- Note that the amount of food the child is able to eat may be insufficient to trigger the response
- If the child has delayed gastric emptying, a delayed gastrocolonic response is produced
- Since colonic inflammation is associated with abnormal motility, it is important to determine if colitis is present. In the case of inflammation, the motility study cannot be interpreted since any abnormality observed may be due to either a primary motility abnormality of the inflammation.

9.5 Anorectal manometry

Indications
- Constipation (including diseases such as Hirschsprung's disease, anismus)
- Fecal incontinence
- To evaluate if medical intervention, surgery, or biofeedback is necessary in patients with the above problems.

Equipment
- Anorectal motility probe (small balloon probe or pediatric water-perfused or solid state anorectal catheter)
- Polygraf
- Perfusion pump, external pressure transducers (not needed if solid state catheter is used)
- Computer
- Analysis software
- Lubricating gel
- 4 × 4 gauzes
- Gloves
- Towels and washcloth
- Three-way stopcocks if water-perfused system is used.

Before the study
- A complete clearance of the lower bowel is needed. Bowel preparations should not be performed for very sick newborns. However, this may cause false-positive results in patients with symptoms that suggest Hirschsprung's disease
- Explain the procedure to the child and the parents
- Sedation of the child should not be necessary. If needed to calm the child, let infants suck on a pacifier or drink from a bottle
- Let parents distract their older children by reading stories to them
- If needed, wait to perform the study until the child falls asleep
- Obtain patient data from parents: symptoms, allergies, and past treatments.

Procedure
As in the adult there are six important parameters to study:
1 maximal voluntary squeeze pressure (external anal sphincter and puborectal muscle function)
2 push/strain pressures
3 rest/relax pressures
4 internal anal sphincter inhibitory response to rectal distention (RAIR)
5 the rectal volume sensory thresholds. The threshold of first sensation (the ability to sense small volumes of rectal distention), to the threshold of maximum tolerable distention

6 defecation dynamics.

For step-by-step instructions, see Section 8.10.

SOME CONSIDERATIONS FOR PEDIATRIC ANORECTAL MANOMETRY

Rectoanal inhibitory reflex

To evaluate the RAIR, the rectal balloon is inflated with 5 ml air or water at body temperature. Withdraw air or water completely within 3–5 s of inflation. Indicate the presence or absence of RAIR, inflated volume and if the child sensed the balloon. Repeat the procedure and increase the inflation with 5–10 ml each time. In infants, volumes up to 30 ml are used. In newborns, a volume of 15 ml is enough to obtain the RAIR.

Defecation dynamics

These can be studied by:

- evaluating the combined external and internal anal sphincter pressures, the external electromyograph (EMG), and the abdominal pressure exerted on the rectum during attempts to defecate
- evaluating the ability to defecate an object from the rectum. Children older than 5 years are asked to defecate a rectal balloon filled with 100 ml water, while sitting on a portable toilet chair. In a healthy child, the balloon is evacuated within the first minute. The defecation effort is evaluated by measuring the highest intraabdominal pressure generated (intraabdominal pressure on the balloon is recorded) and the duration of the straining effort
- Saline continence test: saline at 37°C is infused in the rectum through a small 8 French (F) feeding tube or Dent sleeve device. The open tip is positioned 10 cm above the anal verge. Infusion rate is 60 ml/min up to 240 ml. The child sits upright, and the volume of leakage is determined. Measurement is taken of the volume infused into the rectum when 10 ml or more saline first leaks. If no leakage occurs, the child is instructed to retain the saline for 5 min. Children with weak external anal sphincter function leak as soon as saline infusion starts.

Interpretations

FUNCTIONAL FECAL RETENTION—MAY CAUSE MEGARECTUM

- Impaired rectal and sigmoid sensation to balloon distention
- Decreased spontaneous rectal and sigmoid motility
- Decreased or no rectal contractility induced by rectal distention
- In approximately 50% of these patients, the external anal sphincter and pelvic floor muscles are contracted abnormally during straining. This syndrome is called the spastic pelvic syndrome or anismus
- Threshold volume for rectosphincteric response to distention is increased
- The complete inhibition of the internal and external anal sphincters requires increased distention of the rectum

9

chapter

- In many patients with functional retention, relaxation of the internal and the external anal sphincter occurs before feces is perceived in the rectum.

HIRSCHSPRUNG'S DISEASE (Fig. 9.9)
- RAIR is absent
- Decreased rectal elasticity.

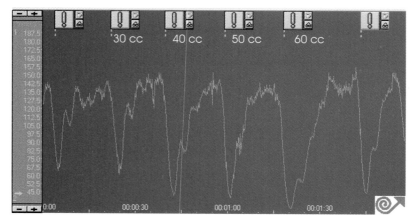

(a)

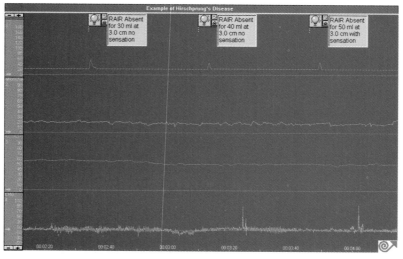

(b)

Figure 9.9 Anorectal manometry in (a) a healthy child and (b) a child with Hirschsprung's disease. (a) The tracing shows a normal RAIR caused by distention with a rectal balloon. Each marking on the tracing shows balloon distention. Increased distention volume causes increased RAIR. (b) Rectal distention from a balloon does not elicit the RAIR in the child with Hirschsprung's disease.

chapter **9**

Pitfalls

It is difficult to use anorectal manometry in the neonatal period when rhythmic activity is absent or anal pressure is low.

9.6 Biofeedback training

Biofeedback training can easily be performed as a fun game for the child. The child tries to copy different curves seen on the monitor and usually only a few training sessions are needed to obtain good results.

There are four conditions that must exist for biofeedback to be successful:
1 a motivated patient
2 a measurable response of the external anal sphincter (contraction or relaxation)
3 the end organ must be capable of responding (e.g. a completely paralyzed, denervated external anal muscle would not respond during biofeedback)
4 the patient must be able to perceive a rectal distention which signals the patient to initiate control.

Indications

- Constipation due to anismus
- Fecal incontinence due to
  (a) weak external anal sphincter (see Fig. 9.11)
  (b) impaired discrimination of rectal sensations
  (c) no synchrony between internal and external anal sphincter response to rectal distention.

Equipment

See Section 8.12.

Procedure

See Section 8.12, and Fig. 9.10.

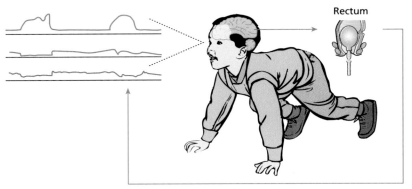

Rectum

Figure 9.10 Biofeedback technique. The child watches the tracings from a healthy individual and is told to attempt to copy the curves seen on the monitor.

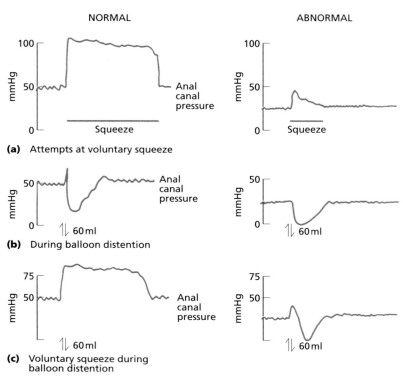

Figure 9.11 Pressure recordings from the anal canal in a child with a weak external anal sphincter compared to a healthy child. The affected child can only accomplish a weak and short voluntary contraction of the external anal sphincter, has no reflex contraction of the external anal sphincter after balloon distention and is unable to override the reflex relaxation when told to squeeze as soon as rectal distention is perceived. Reproduced with permission from Hyman, 1994. Published by Academy Professional Information Services, Inc.

Bibliography

Abell TL, Camilleri M, Hench VS, *et al*. Gastric electromechanical function and gastric emptying in diabetic gastroparesis. *Eur J Gastroenterol Hepatol* 1991; 3: 163–7.

Allen CJ, *et al*. Gastroesophageal reflux and chronic respiratory disease. In: Baum GL, Wolinski E, eds. *Textbook of Pulmonary Diseases*, vol. 2. Boston: Little, Brown, 1989: 1471.

Ashraf W, Wszolek Z, Pfeiffer RF, *et al*. Anorectal function in fluctuating (on–off) Parkinson's disease: evaluation by combined anorectal manometry and electromyography. *Movement Dis* 1995; 10.

Ashraf W, Park F, Lof J, Quigley EMM. An examination of the reliability of reported stool frequency in the diagnosis of idiopathic constipation. *Am J Gastroenterol* 1996; 91(1): 26–32.

Bain WM, Harrington JW, Thomas LE, Schaefer SD. Head and neck manifestations of gastroesophageal reflux. *Laryngoscope* 1983; 93: 175–9.

Baldi F, Ferrarini F, Longanesi A, *et al*. Acid gastroesophageal reflux and symptom occurrence. *Dig Dis Sci* 1987; 34: 1890–3.

Barish CF, Wu WC. Complications of GE-reflux. In: Castell DO, Wu WC, Ott DJ, eds. *Gastroesophageal Reflux Disease*. Mount Kisco, New York: Futura, 1985: 281.

Barish CF, Wu WC, Castell DO. Respiratory complications of gastroesophageal reflux. *Arch Intern Med* 1985; 145: 1882.

Bechi P, Pucciani F, Cosi F, *et al*. Long-term ambulatory enterogastric reflux monitoring. Validation of a new fiberoptic technique. *Dig Dis Sci* 1993; 38: 1297–306.

Benjamin SB, Castell DO. The 'nutcracker esophagus' and the spectrum of esophageal motor disorders. *Curr Concepts Gastroenterol* 1980; 5: 3.

Boix-Ochoa J, Canals J. Maturation of the lower esophagus. *J Pediatr Surg* 1976; 11: 749–56.

Bonavina L, Evander A, DeMeester TR, Walther B, Cheng SC, Palazzo L, Concannon JL. Length of the distal esophageal sphincter and competency of the cardia. *Am J Surg* 1986; 151: 25–34.

BIBLIOGRAPHY

Boyle JT, Cohen S, Watkins JB. Successful treatment of achalasia in childhood by pneumatic dilation. *J Pediatr* 1981; 99: 35–40.

Boyle JT. Pathogenic gastroesophageal reflux in infants and children. *Pract Gastroenterol* 1990; 14: 25–38.

Brand DL, Martin D, Pope CE. Esophageal manometrics in patients with anginal type chest pain. *Am J Dig Dis* 1977; 23: 300.

Bremner RM, Hoeft SF, Constantini M, Crookes PF, Bremner CG, DeMeester TR. Pharyngeal swallowing: the major factor in clearance of esophageal reflux episodes. *Ann Surg* 1993; 218: 364–70.

Burden WR, Hodges RP, Hsu M, O'Leary JP. Alkaline reflux gastritis. *Surg Clin N Am* 1991; 71: 33–44.

Camilleri M, Thompson DG, Malagelada J-R. Functional dyspepsia. Symptoms and underlying mechanism. *J Clin Gastroenterol* 1986; 8(4): 424–9.

Carrasco E, Larrain A, Galleguillos F. Bronchial asthma and gastroesophageal reflux. *Rev Med Chil* 1982; 110: 527–37.

Castell DO (ed.) *The Esophagus*. New York: Little, Brown & Co, 1992.

Castell JA, Gideon M, Castell DO. Esophagus (Chpt. 9). In: Schuster MM, ed. *Atlas of Gastrointestinal Motility*. London: Williams & Wilkins, 1993: 134–57.

Casten DF. Esophageal hiatal hernia and gastric acid secretion. *Arch Surg* 1964; 88: 255–9.

Champion MC, Orr WC (eds). *Evolving Concepts in Gastrointestinal Motility*. Oxford: Blackwell Science, 1996.

Chen J, McCallum RW. Gastric slow wave abnormalities in patients with gastroparesis. *Am J Gastroenterol* 1992; 87: 477–82.

Cherry J, Margulies SI. Contact ulcer of the larynx. *Laryngoscope* 1968; 78: 1937–40.

Clark GWB, Jamieson JR, Hinder RA, Polishuk PV, DeMeester TR, Gupta N, Cheng SC. The relationship of gastric pH and the emptying of solid, semisolid and liquid meals. *J Gastrointest Mot* 1993; 5: 273–9.

Cook IJ, Dodds WJ, Dantas RO, *et al.* Opening mechanisms of the human upper esophageal sphincter. *Am J Physiol* 1989; 257: G748–59.

Cook IJ, Gabb M, Panagopoulos V, *et al.* Pharyngeal (Zenker's) diverticulum is a disorder of upper esophageal sphincter opening. *Gastroenterol* 1992; 103: 1229–35.

Cook IJ. Cricopharyngeal function and dysfunction. *Dysphagia* 1993; 8: 244–51.

Corazziari E, Funch-Jensen P, Hogan WJ, Tanaka M, Toouli J. Functional disorders of the biliary tract. *Gastroenterol Int* 1993; 6(3): 129–44.

Cucchiara S, Bortolotti M, Minella R, Auricchio S. Fasting and postprandial mechanisms of gastroesophageal reflux in children with gastroesophageal reflux disease. *Dig Dis Sci* 1993; 38: 86–92.

Cucchiara S, Minella R, D'Armiento F, Franco MT. *Eur J Gastroenterol Hepatol* 1993; 5: 621–6.

Dantas RO, Cook IJ, Dodds WJ, Kern MK, Lang IM, Brasseur JG. Biomechanics of cricopharyngeal bars. *Gastroenterol* 1990; 99: 1269–74.

Decaestecker JS, Heading RC. Esophageal pH monitoring. *Gastroenterol Clin N Am* 1990; 19: 645–9.

DeMeester TR, O'Sullivan GC, Bermudez G, *et al*. Esophageal function in patients with angina-type chest pain and normal coronary angiograms. *Ann Surg* 1982; 196: 488–98.

DeMeester TR. Definition, detection and pathophysiology of gastroesophageal reflux disease. In: DeMeester TR, Matthews HR, eds. *International Trends in General Thoracic Surgery*. St Louis: Mosby, 1987: vol. 3, 99–127.

DeMeester TR. Prolonged oesophageal pH-monitoring. In: Read NW, ed. *Gastro-intestinal Motility: Which Test?* Petersfield: Wrightson Biomedical Publishing Ltd, 1989: 41–51.

DeMeester TR, Stein HJ, Fuchs KH. Diagnostic studies in the evaluation of the esophagus: physiologic diagnostic studies. In: Orringer MB, ed. *Shackleford's Surgery of the Alimentary Tract*, 3rd edn. Philadelphia: WB Saunders, 1991: 94–126.

Dent J, Dodds WJ, Friedman RH, *et al*. Mechanism of gastroesophageal reflux in recumbent asymptomatic human subjects. *J Clin Invest* 1980; 65: 256–67.

Dent J, Holloway RH, Toouli J, Dodds WJ. Mechanisms of lower oesophageal sphincter incompetence in patients with symptomatic gastroesophageal reflux. *Gut* 1988; 29: 1020–8.

Dixon MF. Progress in pathology of gastritis and duodenitis. In: Williams, GT, ed. *Current Topics in Pathology*. Berlin: Springer-Verlag, 1990: 1–39.

Dodds WJ, Dent J, Hogan WJ, *et al*. Mechanisms of gastroesophageal reflux in patients with reflux esophagitis. *N Engl J Med* 1982; 307: 1547–52.

Dubois A. Role of gastric factors in the pathogenesis of gastroesophageal reflux: emptying, acid, and pepsin, bile reflux. In: Castell DO, Wu WC, Ott DJ, eds. *Gastroesophageal Reflux Disease: Pathogenesis, Diagnosis, Therapy*. Mount Kisco, New York: Futura, 1985: 81–97.

Dubois A, Van Eerdewegh P, Gardner JD. Gastric emptying and secretion in Zollinger–Ellison syndrome. *J Clin Invest* 1977; 59: 255–63.

DuPlessis DJ. Pathogenesis of gastric ulceration. *Lancet* 1965; i: 974–8.

Edwards LL, Quigley EMM, Harned RK, Hofman R, Pfeiffer RF. Characterization of swallowing and defecation in Parkinson's disease. *Am J Gastroenterol* 1994; 89(1): 15–25.

Ellis FH Jr, Schlegel JF, Lynch VP, Payne WS. Cricopharyngeal myotomi for pharyngoesophageal diverticulum. *Ann Surg* 1969; 170: 340–9.

Faulk DL, Anuras S, Christensen J. Chronic intestinal pseudoobstruction. *Gastroenterol* 1978; 74: 922–31.

Fein M, Fuchs KH, Bohrer T, Freys S, Thiede A. Fiberoptic technique for 24 hour bile reflux monitoring—standards and normal values for gastric monitoring. *Dig Dis Sci* 1996; 41(1): 216–25.

Ferguson MK, Little AG. Angina-like chest pain associated with high amplitude peristaltic contractions of the esophagus. *Surgery* 1988; 104: 713–19.

Freys SM, Fuchs KH, Heimbucher J, Beese G, Thiede A. Vektorvolumen-bestimmung des analen sphinkersystems. *Kontinenz* 1993; 2: 67–70.

Fuchs KH, Selch A, Freys SM, DeMeester TR. Gastric acid secretion and gastric pH measurement in peptic ulcer disease. *Prob Gen Surg* 1992; 9: 138–51.

Fuchs KH, Freys SM, Heimbucher J, Fein M, Thiede A. Pathophysiologic spectrum in patients with gastroesophageal reflux disease in a surgical GI function laboratory. *Dis Esoph* 1995; 8: 211–17.

Funch-Jensen P, Kruse A, Ravensbaek J. Endoscopic sphincter of Oddi manometry in healthy volunteers. *Scand J Gastroenterol* 1987; 22: 343.

Funch-Jensen P. Sphincter of Oddi physiology. *J Hep Bil Pancr Surg* 1995; 2: 249–54.

Funch-Jensen P. Defining sphincter of Oddi dysfunction. *Ther Bil Endosc* 1996; 6(1): 1052–57.

Geldof H, Van der Schee EJ, Van Blankenstein M, *et al*. Electrogastro-graphic study of gastric myoelectrical activity in patients with unex-plained nausea and vomiting. *Gut* 1986; 26: 799–808.

Gilles M, Nicks R, Skyring A. Clinical, manometric, and pathologic studies in diffuse esophageal spasm. *Br Med J* 1967; 2: 527.

Goldberg M, Noyek A, Pritzker KPH. Laryngeal granuloma secondary to gastroesophageal reflux. *J Otolaryngol* 1978; 7: 196.

Gotley DC, Morgan AP, Cooper MJ. Bile acid concentrations in the reflux-ate of patients with reflux oesophagitis. *Br J Surg* 1988; 75: 587–90.

Greenfield JL. Pulmonary effects of experimental graded aspiration of hydrochloric acid. *Ann Surg* 1969; 170: 74.

Guelrud M, Mendoza S, Rossiter G, *et al*. Sphincter of Oddi manometry in healthy volunteers. *Dig Dis Sci* 1990; 35: 38–46.

Hallewell JD, Cole TB. Isolated head and neck symptoms due to hiatus hernia. *Arch Otolaryngol* 1970; 92: 499.

Hamberg J, Lindahl O. Angina pectoris symptoms caused by thoracic spine disorders. Clinical examination and treatment. *Acta Med Scand* 1981; Suppl. 644: 84–6.

Harmon JW, Bass BL, Batzri S. Alkaline reflux gastritis. In: Nyhus LL, ed. *Problems in General Surgery*. Philadelphia: Lippincott, 1993: 201–6.

Helm JF, *et al*. The association of heartburn and belching with acid gastroesophageal reflux as assessed by ambulatory pH monitoring. *Gastroenterol* 1988; 94: A182.

Henry RL, Mellis CM. Resolution of inspiratory stridor after fundoplica-tion: case report. *Aust Paediatr J* 1982; 1: 126–7.

Hogan WJ, Viegas de Andrade SR, Winship DH. Ethanol induced acute esophageal motor dysfunction. *J Appl Physiol* 1972; 32: 755–60.

Holland R, Gallagher MD, Quigley EMM. An evaluation of an ambulatory manometry system in assessment of antroduodenal motor activity. *Dig Dis Sci* 1996; 41(8): 1531–7.

Holloway RH, Hongo M, Berger K, McCallum RW. Gastric distention: a mechanism for postprandial gastroesophageal reflux. *Gastroenterol* 1985; 89: 779–84.

Holloway RH, Dent J. Pathophysiology of gastroesophageal reflux. Lower esophageal sphincter dysfunction in gastroesophageal reflux disease. *Gastroenterol Clin N Am* 1990; 19: 517–35.

Hubens A, Van de Kelft E, Roland J. The influence of cholecystectomy on the duodenogastric reflux of bile. *Hepatogastroenterol* 1989; 36: 384–6.

Hyman PE (ed.) *Pediatric Gastrointestinal Motility Disorders*. New York: Academy Professional Information Services Inc., 1994.

Jamieson JR, Stein HJ, DeMeester TR, *et al*. Ambulatory 24 h esophageal pH monitoring: normal values, optimal thresholds, sensitivity, specificity and reproducibility. *Am J Gastroenterol* 1992; 87: 1071–5.

Johansson KE, Ask P, Boeryd B, *et al*. Oesophagitis, signs of reflux and gastric acid secretion in patients with gastro-oesophageal reflux disease. *Scand J Gastroenterol* 1986; 21: 837–47.

Johnson LF, DeMeester TR. 24 hour pH monitoring of the distal esophagus: a quantitative measure of gastro-esophageal reflux. *Am J Gastroenterol* 1974; 62: 325–32.

Kahrilas PJ, Quigley EMM. Clinical esophageal pH recording: a technical review for practice guideline development. *Gastroenterol* 1996; 110: 1982–96.

Kalima TV. Reflux gastritis unrelated to gastric surgery. *Scand J Gastroenterol* 1982; 17 (Suppl. 79): 66–71.

Kiff E, Swash M. Slowed conduction in the pudendal nerves in idiopathic (neurogenic) fecal incontinence. *Br J Surg* 1984; 74: 614–16.

Kiff ES, Barnes RPH, Swash M. Evidence of pudendal nerve neuropathy in patients with perineal descent and chronic straining at stool. *Gut* 1984; 25: 1279–82.

Kilpatrick ZM, Milles SS. Achalasia in mother and daughter. *Gastroenterol* 1972; 62: 1042–6.

Kjellen G, Tibbling L, Wranne B. Bronchial obstruction after oesophageal acid perfusion in asthmatics. *Clin Physiol* 1981: 285–92.

Knuff TE, Benjamin SB, Castell DO. Pharyngoesophageal (Zenker's) diverticulum: a reappraisal. *Gastroenterol* 1982; 82: 734.

Koch KL, Stern RM, Stewart WR, *et al*. Gastric emptying and gastric myoelectrical activity in patients with diabetic gastroparesis: effect of long-term domperidone treatment. *Am J Gastroenterol* 1989; 84: 1069–75.

Koufman JA, *et al*. Reflux laryngitis and its sequellae: the diagnostic role of ambulatory 24-hour pH monitoring. *J Voice* 1988; 2: 78.

BIBLIOGRAPHY

Krishnamurthy S, Schuffler MD. Pathology of neuromuscular disorders of the small intestine and colon. *Gastroenterol* 1987; 93: 610–39.

Kuriloff DB, *et al*. Detection of gastroesophageal reflux in the head and neck: the role of scintigraphy. *Ann Otol Rhinol Laryngol* 1987; 96: 387.

Latimer P, Sarna S, Campbell D, Latimer M, Waterfall W, Daniel EE. Colonic motor and myoelectric activity: a comparative study of normal subjects, psychoneurotic patients, and patients with irritable bowel syndrome. *Gastroenterol* 1981; 80: 893–901.

Levine MD. Children with encopresis: a descriptive analysis. *Pediatrics* 1975; 56: 412–16.

Loening Baucke VA. Sensitivity of the sigmoid colon and rectum in children treated for chronic constipation. *J Pediatr Gastroenterol Nutr* 1984; 3: 454–9.

Loening-Baucke VA. Factors determining outcome in children with chronic constipation and faecal soiling. *Gut* 1989; 30: 999–1006.

London FA, Raab DE, Fuller J. Achalasia in three siblings: a rare occurrence. *Mayo Clin Proc* 1977; 52: 97–100.

Mackler D, Schneider R. Achalasia in father and son. *Am J Dig Dis* 1978; 23: 1042–5.

Malagelada J-R, Stanghellini V. Manometric evaluation of functional upper gut symptoms. *Gastroenterol* 1985; 88: 1223–31.

Malagelada J-R. *Manometric Diagnosis of Gastrointestinal Motility Disorders*. New York: Thieme, 1986.

Malagelada J-R, Camilleri M, Stanghellini V. *Manometric Diagnosis of Gastrointestinal Motility Disorder*. New York: Thieme, 1986.

Mansfield LE, Stein MR. GE reflux and asthma: a possible reflex mechanism. *Ann Allergy* 1978; 41: 224.

McKee D, Quigley EMM. Intestinal motility in irritable bowel syndrome: is IBS a motility disorder? Part I: Definition of IBS and colonic motility. *Dig Dis Sci* 1993; 38(10): 1761–72.

McKee D, Quigley EMM. Intestinal motility in irritable bowel syndrome: is IBS a motility disorder? Part 2: Motility of small bowel, esophagus, stomach, and gall-bladder. *Dig Dis Sci* 1993; 38(10): 1773–82.

McNally PR, Maydonovitch CL, Prosek RA, Collette RP, Wong RK. Evaluation of gastroesophageal reflux as a cause of idiopathic hoarseness. *Dig Dis Sci* 1989; 34: 1900–4.

Mela GS, Savarino V, Malesci A, Di Mario F, Sossai P, Vigneri S, Zambotti A. New method for improving accuracy of 24-hour continuous intragastric pH-metry. Reflections on physiological and pharmacological studies. *Dig Dis Sci* 1994; 39: 1416–24.

Meyer W, Vollmar F, Bar W. Barrett esophagus following total gastrectomy. A contribution to its pathogenesis. *Endoscopy* 1979; 11: 121–6.

Miko TL. Peptic (contact ulcer) granuloma of the larynx. *J Clin Pathol* 1989; 42: 800–4.

Milla P (ed.) *Disorders of Gastrointestinal Motility in Childhood.* New York: John Wiley & Sons, 1988.

Misiewicz JJ, Waller SL, Anthony PP, Gummer JW. Achalasia of the cardia: pharmacology and histopathology of isolated cardiac sphincteric muscle from patients with and without achalasia. *Q J Med* 1969; 38: 17–30.

Mittal RK, McCallum RW. Characteristics of transient lower esophageal sphincter relaxation in humans. *Am J Physiol* 1987; 252: G636–41.

Mittal RK, McCallum RW. Characteristics and frequency of transient relaxations of the lower esophageal sphincter on patients with reflux esophagitis. *Gastroenterol* 1988; 95: 593–9.

Mittal RK, Lange RC, McCallum RW. Identification and mechanism of delayed acid clearance in subjects with hiatus hernia. *Gastroenterol* 1987; 92: 130–5.

Mittal RK, Rochester DF, McCallum RW. Effect of the diaphragmatic contraction on lower esophageal sphincter pressure in man. *Gut* 1987; 28: 1564–8.

Morrison MD. Is chronic gastroesophageal reflux a causative factor in glottic carcinoma? *Otolaryngol Head Neck Surg* 1988; 99: 370.

Muller-Lissner SA, Schindlbeck NE, Heinrich C. Bile salt reflux after cholecystectomy. *Scand J Gastroenterol* 1987; 22 (Suppl. 139): 20–4.

Nagler RW, *et al.* Achalasia in fraternal twins. *Ann Intern Med* 1963; 59: 906.

Nano M, Palmas F, Giaccone M, *et al.* Biliary reflux after cholecystectomy: a prospective study. *Hepatogastroenterol* 1990; 37: 233–4.

Orenstein SR. Effects on behavior state of prone versus seated positioning for infants with gastroesophageal reflux. *Pediatrics* 1990; 85: 765–7.

Ossakow SJ, Elta G, Colturi T, Bogdasarian R, Nostrant TT. Esophageal reflux and dysmotility as the basis for persistent cervical symptoms. *Ann Otol Rhinol Laryngol* 1987; 96: 387–92.

Pellegrini CA, DeMeester TR, Johnson LF, Skinner DB. Gastroesophageal reflux and pulmonary aspiration: incidence, functional abnormality and results of surgical therapy. *Surgery* 1979; 86: 110–19.

Preston DM, Lennard-Jones JE. Anismus in chronic constipation. *Dig Dis Sci* 1985; 30: 413–18.

Quigley EMM. Small intestinal motor activity—its role in gut homeostasis in health and disease. *Q J Med* 1987; 65: 799–810.

Quigley EMM. Gastroesophageal reflux disease: the roles of motility in pathophysiology and therapy. Editorials. *Am J Gastroenterol* 1993; 88(10): 1649–51.

Quigley EMM. Intestinal manometry in man: a historical and clinical perspective. *Dig Dis* 1994; 12: 199–209.

Quigley EMM. Epidemiology and pathophysiology of gastrointestinal manifestations in Parkinson's disease. In: Corazziari E, ed. *Neurogastroenterology.* Berlin: Walter de Gruyter, 1996: 168–78.

Quigley EMM. Gastric and small intestinal motility in health and disease. *Gastrointest Motility Clin Prac* 1996; 25(1): 113–145.

Read NW, Timms JM, Barfield LJ, Donnelly TC, Bannister JJ. Impairment of defecation in young women with severe constipation. *Gastroenterol* 1986; 90: 53–60.

Ritchie WP. Alkaline reflux gastritis: an objective assessment of its diagnosis and treatment. *Ann Surg* 1980; 92: 288–98.

Ritchie WP. Alkaline reflux gastritis: late results on a controlled trial of diagnosis and treatment. *Ann Surg* 1986; 203: 537–44.

Robertson CS, Martin BAB, Atkinson M. Possible role of herpes viruses in the etiology of achalasia of the cardia. *Gut* 1989; 30: A731.

Sataloff RT. Professional singers: the science and art of clinical care. *Am J Otolaryngol* 1981; 2: 251.

Schuffler MD. Chronic intestinal pseudoobstruction syndromes. *Med Clin N Am* 1981; 65: 1331–58.

Schuffler MD, Rohrmann CA, Chaffee RG, Grand DL, Delaney JH, Young JH. Chronic intestinal pseudo-obstruction: a report of 27 cases and review of the literature. *Medicine* 1981; 60: 173–96.

Schuster MM (ed.) *Atlas of Gastrointestinal Motility in Health and Disease*. London: Williams & Wilkins, 1993.

Smout AJPM. *Normal and Disturbed Motility of the Gastrointestinal Tract*. Petersfield, Wrightson Biomedical Publishing Ltd, 1992.

Snooks SJ, Barnes RPH, Swash M. Damage to the voluntary anal and urinary sphincter musculative in incontinence. *J Neurol Neurosurg Psychiatry* 1984; 47: 1269–73.

Snooks SJ, Swash M. Nerve stimulation techniques. In: Henry MM, Swash M, eds. *Coloproctology and the Pelvic Floor: Pathophysiology and Management*. London: Butterworths, 1985.

Sontag SJ, O'Connell S, Khandelwal S, *et al*. Most asthmatics have gastro-esophageal reflux with or without bronchodilator therapy. *Gastroenterol* 1990; 99: 613–20.

Stanghellini V, Camilleri M, Malagelada JR. Chronic idiopathic intestinal pseudoobstruction: clinical and intestinal manometric findings. *Gut* 1987; 28: 5–12.

Stein JH, DeMeester TR, Naspetti R. Three dimensional imaging of the lower esophageal sphincter in gastroesophageal reflux disease. *Ann Surg* 1991; 214: 374–84.

Stein JH, DeMeester TR. Indications, technique, and clinical use of ambulatory 24-hour esophageal motility monitoring. *Ann Surg* 1993; 217: 128–37.

Stein JH, DeMeester TR, Peters JH, Fuchs KH. Technique, indications, and clinical use of ambulatory 24-hour gastric monitoring in a surgical practice. *Surgery* 1994; 116: 758–67.

Talley NJ, McNeil D, Hayden A, Piper DW. Randomized double-blind placebo controlled crossover trial of cimetidine and pirenzepine in non-ulcer dyspepsia. *Gastroenterol* 1986; 91: 149–56.

Teisanu E, Hociota D, Dimitriu T, Marcu P, Calarasu R, Marinescu A. Pharyngolaryngeal disturbances in patients with gastroesophageal reflux. *Rev Chir Oncol Radiol O R L Oftalmol Stomatol Otorhinolaryngol* 1978; 23: 279–86.

Telander RL, Morgan KG, Kreulen DL, Schmalz PF, Kelly KA, Szurszewski JH. Human gastric atony with tachygastria and gastric retention. *Gastroenterol* 1978; 75: 497–501.

Toouli J, Roberts-Thomson IC, Dent J, Lee J. Manometric disorders in patients with suspected sphincter of Oddi dysfunction. *Gastroenterol* 1985; 88: 1243–50.

Vaezi MF, Richter JE. Complicated Barrett's esophagus. Role of acid and bile. *Ann J Gastroenterol* 1994; 89: 1630 (Abstr.).

Vaezi MF, LaCamera RG, Richter JE. Bilitec 2000 ambulatory duodeno-gastric reflux monitoring system. Studies on its validation and limitations. *Am J Physiol* 1994; 267: G1050–7.

Vandenplas Y, Goyvaerts H, Helven R, Sacre L. Gastroesophageal reflux, as assessed by 24 hour pH monitoring, in 509 healthy infants screened for SIDS-risk. *Pediatrics* 1991; 88: 834–40.

Vandenplas Y, Belli D, Boige N, et al. A standardized protocol for the methodology of esophageal pH monitoring and interpretation of the data for the diagnosis of gastro-esophageal reflux. *J Pediatr Gastroenterol Nutr* 1992; 14: 467–71.

von Leden H, Moore P. Contact ulcer of the larynx. Experimental observations. *Arch Otolaryngol* 1960; 72: 746.

Wald A, Chandra R, Chiponis D, Gabel S. Anorectal function and continence mechanisms in childhood encopresis. *J Pediatr Gastroenterol Nutr* 1986; 5: 346–51.

Walther B, DeMeester TR. Placement of the esophageal pH electrode for 24 hour esophageal pH monitoring. In: DeMeester TR, Skinner DB, eds. *Esophageal Disorders: Pathophysiology and Therapy*. New York: Raven Press, 1985: 539.

Ward PH, Berci G. Observations on the pathogenesis of chronic non-specific pharyngitis and laryngitis. *Laryngoscope* 1982; 92: 1377.

Ward PH, Ippoliti AF, Simmons DH, Maloney JV Jr. Specialty conference: complications of gastroesophageal reflux. *West J Med* 1988; 149: 58–65.

Whitehead WE, Holtkotter B, Enck P, et al. Tolerance for rectosigmoid distension in irritable bowel syndrome. *Gastroenterol* 1990; 98: 1187–92.

Wilson P, Perdikis G, Hinder RA, Redmond EJ, Anselmino M, Quigley EM. Prolonged ambulatory antroduodenal manometry in humans. *Am J Gastroenterol* 1994; 89(9): 1489–95.

Wright RA, Miller SA, Corsello BF. Acid induced esophago-bronchial-cardiac reflexes in humans. *Gastroenterol* 1990; 99: 71–3.

BIBLIOGRAPHY

Zaninotto G, DeMeester TR. Gastroesophageal reflux disease. In: Kumar D, Gustavsson S, eds. *An Illustrated Guide to Gastrointestinal Motility*. New York: John Wiley, 1988: 324–34.

Index

277